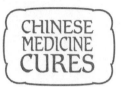

CHINESE
MEDICINE
CURES

ARTHRITIS

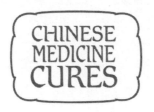

ARTHRITIS

BOB FLAWS & DOUGLAS FRANK

Adapted for the UK by Sylvia Schroer

foulsham
LONDON • NEW YORK • TORONTO • SYDNEY

foulsham

The Publishing House, Bennetts Close, Cippenham,
Slough, Berkshire, SL1 5AP, England

ISBN 0–572–02540-8

Typeset by Grafica, Bournemouth
Printed in Great Britain by St. Edmundsbury Press, Bury St. Edmunds, Suffolk

CONTENTS

INTRODUCTION

WHAT IS ARTHRITIS?

Arthritis means joint (*arthr-*) inflammation (*-itis*). When prefaced by the word osteo, it simply means inflammation of the joints of the bones. Other names for osteoarthritis (OA) are degenerative joint disease (DJD), osteoarthroses (*i.e.*, bone joint condition), and hypertrophic osteoarthritis. It is the most common of all forms of joint disease, typically first appearing asymptomatically in the 20s and 30s and becoming universal by age 70. As the authors of *The Merck Manual*, one of the 'bibles' of Western doctors, says, 'Almost all persons by age 40 have some pathologic changes in the weight-bearing joints, although relatively few people are symptomatic [by that age].'[1]

Rheumatoid arthritis (RA) is by far the most serious, painful and potentially crippling form of arthritis. It is a chronic systemic disease characterised by flare-ups and remissions. Rheumatoid arthritis primarily attacks the joints but may affect the supporting connective tissues throughout the body, causing fever, weakness, fatigue, and deformity. The trigger of RA is unknown although there is speculation about viruses, environmental agents and the involvement of genetic factors. RA is an auto-immune process whereby auto-antibodies which are generated by the body act against structural elements with the joints.

---

[1] *The Merck Manual of Diagnosis and Therapy*, 15th edition, ed. by Robert Berkow, Merck Sharp & Dohme Research Laboratories, Rahway, NJ, 1987, p.1258

Other types of arthritis include spondyloarthropatries, *e.g.* anklylosing spondylitis, arthritis associated with infections or illnesses, *e.g.* psoriatic arthritis, and infective or sceptic arthritis.

WHO GETS ARTHRITIS?

While both men and women get arthritis, the incidence in women is significantly higher — about two to one. However, its onset is typically earlier in men than in women. Osteoarthritis is found in all climates throughout the world. In fact, OA occurs in almost all vertebrates. The only two mammals it does not occur in are bats and sloths which both spend much of their lives hanging upside down! OA is more likely to be associated with old age, whilst RA occurs through adult life. Sceptic arthritis is seen in children and its symptoms and onset can be very extreme.

WHAT CAUSES ARTHRITIS?

The cause of arthritis according to modern Western medicine depends on the type of arthritis it is. OA is basically caused by wear and tear, whilst other types of arthritis may involve the immune process. Some factors which may contribute to the onset of arthritis are congenital joint abnormalities, genetic defects, infectious, metabolic, endocrine and neuropathic diseases, virtually any disease which alters the normal structure and function of the cartilage covering the inner surfaces of the joint, and acute and chronic trauma affecting this cartilage. In terms of this last cause, we are talking about wear and tear. Any motion which repeatedly puts stress on the inner surfaces of the joint may result in micro-trauma leading eventually to inflammation. When this kind of micro-trauma continues year after year, as in certain occupations such as foundry workers and bus drivers, a whole series of micro-traumas sooner or later adds up to significant damage to the surfaces of the joints. Whether this happens sooner or later often depends on other factors affecting our health, such as our metabolism, our hormones, our immune system, and various infectious diseases.

WHAT ARE THE SIGNS AND SYMPTOMS OF ARTHRITIS?

With the exception of sceptic arthritis in children, the onset of arthritis is usually subtle and gradual and begins by affecting only one or two joints. Its first symptom is pain and this pain is typically made worse by exercise. Different types of arthritis typically affect different joints. OA affects weight-bearing joints, such as the knees and hips. RA often affects the hands. Spondyloarthropatries affects the back and axial skeleton, including the shoulders and hip girdle. Gout affects the big toe and may affect the ankles and knees – white depositis known as trophi may show with this condition. Basically, OA becomes worse later in the day, whilst RA starts off badly early on but improves as the day goes on. As the disease progresses, joint mobility becomes diminished and flexion contractures occur. One may hear a grating noise and feel a grating sensation within the joint when it is moved. This is called crepitus. Eventually, the affected joints become enlarged and may even become hot to the touch and red in colour. As the ligaments holding the joint in place become lax, the joint may become increasingly unstable and increasingly painful. Tenderness on palpation around the affected joint and pain on passive motion (*i.e.*, when someone else moves the joint for you) are late signs in the progression of this disease. Adding insult to injury, muscular spasms add to the pain. Eventually, as the inflammatory process continues to affect the cartilage and underlying bone tissue, the joint may become deformed, the surrounding muscles may atrophy, and nodular pseudocysts may appear.

HOW DOES WESTERN MEDICINE
DIAGNOSE ARTHRITIS?

The Western medical diagnosis of arthritis is usually based on the above signs and symptoms. X-rays are very important. With RA, a test may be done for Rheumatoid Factor. Gout may be detected by looking at uric acid levels. Sometimes a test for blood sedimentation rates is done, which thus confirms the presence of an inflammatory process.

HOW DOES WESTERN MEDICINE
TREAT ARTHRITIS?

The Western medical treatment of arthritis depends on the type of arthritis. Non-steroidal anti-inflammatories (NSAIDS) are frequently given for pain relief, for example aspirin, ibuprofen, indomethacin and voltarol or diclofenac. A curious anomaly regarding NSAIDs has been highlighted by Dr Jason Theodosakis:

> What's curious is that while these drug companies come out with new versions of the same thing, an anti-inflammatory agent, osteoarthritis is mostly non-inflammatory. Only occasionally do you find inflammation in the later stages of the disease. Furthermore, there is some preliminary evidence that when you put anti-inflammatory pills in a culture with cartilage cells, it impairs the healing process. So you're covering up the pain but probably impairing the healing process and stopping the signals that you have joint pain... they do not address the cause of the disease and may in fact worsen it.[3]

One of the effects of NSAIDs and aspirin usage not commonly mentioned in the medical literature, such as *The Merck Manual*, is that they impair cartilage repair. In fact, NSAIDs and aspirin usage has been linked to *increased cartilage destruction!*[3] This side effect is ironic since most users of nsaids and aspirin are people with osteoarthritis caused by cartilage damage in the first place. Dr. Theodosakis goes on to say that, 'When you give people anti-inflammatory pills, even in the highest doses, only 70 per cent get pain relief.'[4]

Unfortunately, the use of NSAIDs also often has side-effects. The most common side-effect is gastrointestinal irritation and ulceration. One study found that one-third of bleeding ulcers in people over 60 years of age is due to aspirin and NSAIDs.[5] The long-term use of NSAIDs is controversial even within Western medicine. Other pain relieving drugs include those that contain codeine, *e.g.* dyhydrocodeine, codydramol and cocodamol. Distalgesic may also be given which contains coproxamol. This is related to codeine. Codeine is an addictive substance and causes constipation.

The more powerful medications for arthritic diseases have even more powerful side-effects. Corticosteroids, such as prednisone used in the treatment of rheumatoid and psioratic arthritis, suppress the immune system. Long-term usage of corticosteroids has been correlated to increased incidence of bone fractures and cataracts.[5] Other treatments for RA include anti-malarials, gold injections and even immune suppressing drugs such as azathiaprine. All these treatments have significant side-effects, including skin reactions, gastrointestinal upset, hepatoxicity and jaundice. Methotrexate, an immune suppresser, may cause bone marrow failure.

Many of the drugs used in the treatment of the arthritic diseases interfere with the absorption of vitamins and minerals in the body. So not only are these medications adversely

_____

[3] Theodosakis, Jason, 'The Amazing Cure for Arthritis: An interview with Jason Theodosakis, M.D., M.S., M.H.P.', *Nexus, Colorado's Holistic Journal,* Boulder, CO, May/June 1997, p. 27

[4] *Ibid.*, p. 30

[5] Ronco, P., and Flahault, A., 'A Drug-induced End Stage Renal Disease', *New England Journal of Medicine,* Vol. 331, No. 25, 1994, pp. 1711-1712

affecting various systems of the body, but they are also robbing the body of its essential nutritional building blocks for health and recovery.

Surgery, including laminectomy of the spine and total joint replacement (as of the hip), are sometimes also resorted to when all other therapy has failed.

WHAT DOES CHINESE MEDICINE HAVE TO OFFER SUFFERERS FROM ARTHRITIS?

Chinese medicine has two main things to offer sufferers of arthritis. The first is a whole range of natural treatments which help relieve pain but also promote healing of the tissues of the joints. These treatments include professionally prescribed and administered acupuncture and moxibustion, Chinese medical massage, and Chinese herbal medicine taken internally and used externally on the affected area. In addition, there are a number of highly effective, time-tested Chinese home remedies and self-treatments for joint pain.

Secondly, Chinese medicine has a much more down-to-earth and immediately understandable vision of what causes joint pain and what you can do for it. Most of us, on hearing that the most probable initial event in OA is the mitosis of the chondrocyte with increased synthesis of proteoglycans and type II collagen, won't have the faintest notion of what this means, or what we ourselves can do about it. Traditional Chinese medicine, on the other hand, is based on a vision of the human body as a microcosmic miniature of the natural world. Therefore, the language of Chinese medicine is the language we use every day to describe events in the world around us. By using this language we are better able to understand our condition and enabled to take charge of our own lives and well-being.

So now, let's turn to how Chinese medicine describes and treats joint pain.

BASIC CONCEPTS
OF CHINESE MEDICINE

The Chinese medical term for all rheumatic diseases, including all types of arthritis, is *bi zheng*. This translates as 'impediment condition'. In Chinese medicine, *bi* or impediment means a blockage or obstruction that results in pain. A number of questions come to mind from this statement. What is being blocked or obstructed? How does this blockage or obstruction come about? And, probably the most important question, especially for people suffering with arthritis, what can be done to reduce or eliminate this pain? It is my hope that this book will help you see how Chinese medicine answers these questions.

To understand how traditional Chinese medicine answers the above questions and treats rheumatic *bi* pain, we first need to describe and explain some of the fundamental concepts of this ancient and holistic medical system. As a system, Chinese medicine is logical. Based on its theories, a practitioner can treat many conditions. It is pragmatic and scientific in its own way. Chinese medicine is a separate system from modern Western medicine, and, as such, cannot be explained in terms of Western medical language or logic. In other words, to understand the how and why of Chinese medicine, we need to approach it on its own terms.

On first hearing about the theories and concepts of Chinese medicine, they may seem strange and unfamiliar. However, Chinese medicine has effectively treated millions of people for several thousand years and as such has gained its own credibility, particularly in China where it evolved. Just as we feel Western medicine applies to us, the Chinese are influenced by their system. Should you find any of the language or terms used to describe the concepts of Chinese medicine difficult to understand, there is a glossary at the back of the book to which you can refer.

YIN AND YANG

Yin and yang are the cornerstones for understanding, diagnosing, and treating the body and mind in Chinese medicine. In a sense, all other theories and concepts of Chinese medicine are simply an elaboration of these fundamental concepts. Most people have probably already heard of the terms yin and yang but may not have a clear idea of what they mean.

The concepts of yin and yang can be used to describe everything that exists in the universe, including all the parts and functions of the body. Originally, yin referred to the shady side of a hill and yang to the sunny side of the hill. Since sunshine and shade are two interdependent sides of a single reality, these two aspects of the hill are seen as part of a single whole. Other examples of yin and yang are that night exists only in relation to day and cold exists only in relation to heat. According to Chinese thought, every single thing that exists in the universe has these two aspects, a yin and a yang. Thus every thing has a front and a back, a top and a bottom, a left and a right, and a beginning and an end. However, a thing is yin or yang *only in relation to its paired complement.* Nothing is in itself yin or yang.

It is the concepts of yin and yang that make Chinese medicine a holistic medicine. This is because, based on this unitary and complementary vision of reality, no body part or body function is viewed as separate or isolated from the whole person. The table opposite shows some examples of yin and yang pairs as they apply to the body. It is important to remember that each item listed is neither yin or yang in itself, but only in relation to its complementary partner. Nothing is of itself either yin or yang.

Yin	Yang
form	function
organs	bowels
blood	qi
inside	outside
front of body	back of body
right side	left side
lower body	upper body
cool, cold	warm, hot
stillness	activity, movement

According to Chinese thought all aspects of nature and the universe may be described through the fundamental concepts of yin and yang.

Qi

Qi (pronounced chee) and blood are two of the most important complementary pairs of yin and yang within the human body. It is said that, in the world, yin and yang are water and fire, but, in the human body, yin and yang are blood and qi. Qi is yang in relation to blood which is yin. Qi is often translated as energy and definitely energy is a manifestation of qi. Chinese language scholars would say, however, that qi is larger than any single type of energy described by modern Western science. Paul Unschuld, one of the greatest living sinologists in my opinion, translates the word qi as influences. This conveys the sense that qi is what is responsible for change and movement. Thus, within Chinese medicine, qi is that which motivates all movement and transformation or change.

In Chinese medicine, qi is defined as having five specific functions:

1. Defence

It is qi which is responsible for protecting the exterior of the body from invasion by external pathogens. This qi, called defensive qi, flows through the exterior portion of the body. The defensive qi plays an extremely important role in the development and the prevention of rheumatic *bi* conditions. As we shall see, when this qi is weak, external pathogens can enter and lodge in the body, especially in the joints, creating the blockage and obstruction that then develop into rheumatic *bi* conditions.

2. Transformation

Qi transforms substances so that they can be utilised by the body. An example of this function is the transformation of the food we eat into nutrients to nourish the body, thus producing more qi and blood.

3. Warmth

Qi, being relatively yang, is inherently warm. One of the main functions of the qi is to warm the entire body, both inside and out. If this warming function of the qi is weak, cold may cause the flow of qi and blood to be congealed similarly to the way cold causes water to produce ice.

4. Restraint

It is qi which holds all the organs and substances in their proper place. Thus all the organs, blood, and fluids need qi to keep them from falling or leaking out of their specific pathways. If this function of qi is weak, then problems like uterine prolapse, easy bruising, or urinary incontinence may occur.

5. Transportation

Qi provides the motivating force for all transportation in the body. Every aspect of the body that moves is moved by the qi. Hence the qi moves the blood and body fluids throughout the body. It is also qi which moves food through the stomach and the blood through its vessels.

BLOOD

In Chinese medicine, blood refers to the red fluid that flows through our vessels as recognised in modern Western medicine, but it also has meanings and implications which are different. Blood is that substance which nourishes and moistens all the body tissues. Without blood, no body tissue can function properly. If there is an insufficient blood supply the tissues become dry and wither.

Qi and blood are closely interrelated. It is said that, 'Qi is the commander of the blood, and blood is the mother of qi'. This means that it is qi which moves the blood but that it is the blood which provides the nourishment and physical foundation for the creation and existence of the qi.

In Chinese medicine, blood provides the following functions for the body:

1. Nourishment

Blood nourishes the body. Along with qi, the blood goes to every part of the body. If the blood is insufficient, its nourishing function decreases and tissues atrophy or shrink.

2. Moistening

Blood moistens the body tissues. This includes the skin, eyes and ligaments and tendons of the body. Blood insufficiency can cause drying out and consequent stiffening of various tissues throughout the body.

3. Blood provides the material foundation for the spirit or mind

In Chinese medicine, the mind and body are considered as one. The blood (yin) supplies the material support and nourishment for the mind (yang) allowing it to become 'bright' (*i.e.* conscious and clever) and stay rooted in the body. If blood is insufficient, the mind can 'float', causing problems like insomnia, agitation and unrest.

ESSENCE

Along with qi and blood, essence is one of the three most important constituents of the body. Essence is the most fundamental material the body utilises for its growth, maturation and reproduction. There are two forms of this essence. We inherit essence from our parents and we also produce our own essence from the food and drink we consume and the air we breathe.

The essence which comes from our parents is what determines our basic constitution, strength and vitality. We each have a finite, limited amount of this inherited essence. It is important to protect and conserve this essence because all bodily functions depend upon it, and, when it is gone, we die. Thus, the depletion of essence has serious implications for our overall health and well-being. Fortunately, the essence derived from food and drink helps to bolster and support this inherited essence. This is possible if we eat healthily and do not use more of our qi and blood than we create each day. Then, when we sleep at night, the surplus qi and especially the blood are transformed into essence.

THE VISCERA AND BOWELS

In Chinese medicine, the internal organs have a wider area of function and influence than in Western medicine. Each organ has distinct responsibilities for maintaining the physical health and psychological well-being of the individual. When thinking about the internal organs according to Chinese medicine it is more accurate to view an organ as a network that spreads throughout the body, and not as a distinct physical organ as described by Western science. In Chinese medicine, the relationship between the various organs and other parts of the body is made possible by the channel and network vessel system which we will discuss below.

Since the internal organs are conceived differently and perform different functions from their same-named organs in modern Western medicine, they are referred to as the viscera and bowels. There are five main viscera which are considered to be relatively yin and six main bowels which are considered to be relatively yang. The five yin viscera are the heart, lungs, liver, spleen and kidneys. The six yang bowels are the stomach, small intestine, large intestine, gallbladder, urinary bladder and a system that Chinese medicine refers to as the triple burner. All bodily functions may be described by reactions of the viscera and bowels. Chinese medicine *as a system* does not 'have' a pancreas, a pituitary gland or the ovaries. The functions of these Western organs are described within the Chinese medicine system of the viscera and bowels.

The five viscera are vitally important in this system. They are responsible for the creation and transformation of qi and blood and the storage of essence. They each have many individual functions, for example, the kidneys are responsible for the excretion of urine but are also responsible for hearing, the strength of the bones including the low back, sexual reproduction, maturation and growth. So, although the Chinese organs may have the same name and even some overlapping functions, they are quite different from the organs of modern Western medicine. Each of the five viscera also has a corresponding tissue, sense, spirit and emotion related to it. These are outlined in the table below.

ORGAN CORRESPONDENCES

In addition, each viscus or bowel possesses both a yin and a yang aspect. The yin aspect of a viscus or bowel refers to its substantial nature or tangible form. Furthermore, an organ's yin is responsible for the nurturing, cooling and moistening of that viscus or bowel. The yang aspect of the viscus or bowel represents its functional activities or what it does. An organ's yang aspect is also warming. These two aspects, yin and yang, form and function, cooling and heating, create good health when they are in balance. However, an imbalance of yin or yang will result in disease.

Organ	Tissue	Sense	Spirit	Emotion
Kidneys	bones/head hair	hearing	will	fear
Liver	sinews	sight	ethereal soul	anger
Spleen	flesh	taste	thought	obsession/worry
Lungs	skin/body hair	smell	corporeal soul	grief/sadness
Heart	blood vessels	speech	spirit	joy/fright

The health of all five viscera is necessary for the prevention and/or the development of rheumatic *bi* problems, but the viscera most directly concerned with rheumatic *bi* conditions are the kidneys, spleen and liver. The involvement of these three viscera in rheumatic *bi* can serve to illustrate the holistic nature of Chinese medicine. When these three viscera function properly and work together harmoniously, the body does not develop chronic rheumatic *bi* problems. If these three viscera do not function properly, then the body is at risk and may develop acute and, eventually, chronic rheumatic *bi* problems.

The remainder of this chapter will focus on the basic functions of the kidneys, spleen and liver. In the next chapter, we will explore the relationship between these three viscera and the condition of rheumatic *bi*.

The kidneys

In Chinese medicine, the kidneys are considered to be the foundation of human life. Since the developing foetus is shaped like a kidney and because the kidneys are the main organ for the storage of inherited essence, the kidneys are referred to as the prenatal root. It is essential to good health and longevity to keep the kidney qi strong and kidney yin and yang in relative balance. Exercises and lifestyle suggestions to develop, protect, and keep the kidneys 'robust', are discussed in Chapter 10.

The most important Chinese medical aspects relating to the kidneys in terms of joint pain are:

1. The kidneys are responsible for human reproduction, development and maturation. You may notice that these are the same functions we described when we discussed the essence. This is because there is a strong relationship between essence and the kidneys and the essence is said to be stored in the kidneys. Health problems relating to reproduction, development and maturation are commonly problems of kidney essence. Excessive sexual activity, drug use or simply prolonged overexertion can all damage or consume the kidney essence.

2. The kidneys are said to rule the bones and marrow. This function includes the joints. This means that all chronic rheumatic *bi* problems involve the kidneys. Even if the disease did not start out affecting the kidneys, over time, chronic *bi zheng* will inevitably involve the kidneys. In Chinese it is said, 'Enduring diseases will reach the kidneys.' Conditions such as osteoporosis, degenerative disc disease and weak legs and knees also typically point to problems with the kidneys.

3. The kidneys are the foundation of water metabolism. They work in coordination with the lungs and spleen to ensure that water is correctly distributed throughout the body and that excess water is excreted as urination. So problems such as swelling or oedema, excessive dryness or excessive urination can indicate a weakness of kidney function.

4. Kidney yin and yang are said to be the foundation for the yin and yang of all the other organs, bowels and body tissues. In other words, the kidneys are the foundation of our life. If either kidney yin or yang is insufficient, eventually the yin or yang of the other viscera and bowels will also be affected. The clinical implications of this will become more clear when we present rheumatic *bi* case histories.

5. The low back is said to be the 'mansion' of the kidneys. This means that the lower back is very closely related to the health of the kidneys. If the kidneys are weak, then you may suffer with low back pain.

The spleen

The spleen may also be of crucial importance in relation to rheumatic *bi* problems. The spleen and its paired bowel, the stomach, are central in the digestive process. The spleen plays a vital role in the body's ability to transform food and drink into qi and blood. The spleen, kidneys and lungs all play a part in the metabolism and movement of water throughout the body. However, the spleen plays the most crucial part when excessive body fluids gather and collect, transforming into what is known as dampness, such as when the joints are swollen in RA. Those familiar with Western anatomy and physiology may be puzzled as they compare the Chinese medicine ideas of spleen function with those described by Western physiology. This is a good illustration of how Chinese medicine views the internal organs and their functions differently from Western medicine.

Chinese medical concepts which relate to the spleen in terms of joint pain include:

1. The spleen governs the transportation and transformation of food and water. This means that the spleen takes the partially digested food and fluids from the stomach and begins the process of transforming it into qi, blood, and essence. A healthy spleen is vital for producing sufficient qi and blood.

2. The spleen contains the blood. The spleen qi is said to hold the blood within its vessels. Therefore, if there is spleen qi vacuity, or deficiency, the person may experience various types of bleeding disorders or bruise easily.

3. The spleen is said to govern the muscles and the four limbs. The muscles are dependent upon the spleen for their nourishment. If this spleen function is weak, the muscles will be weak and the legs and arms will lack power.

The liver
The liver is the third viscus in Chinese medicine frequently implicated in rheumatic *bi* conditions. While the bones and joints are related to the kidneys, the liver has a strong influence on the joints due to its control over the orderly spreading of the qi and its correspondence with the 'sinews'.

The basic Chinese medical concepts which relate to the liver include the following:

1. The liver is said to control coursing and discharge. Coursing and discharge refer here to the orderly spreading of qi to every part of the body. To be healthy, it is important the qi reaches all over the body. If the liver is not able to maintain the free and smooth flow of qi throughout the body, multiple physical and even emotional symptoms can develop. This vital function of the liver is most easily damaged by emotional causes and, in particular, by stress and frustration. When we are frustrated, our qi wants to flow but the circumstances won't allow it. Usually, we repress our feelings in such instances and this can then result in depression and constraint of the flow of qi controlled by the liver. This type of stagnation and constraint of the flow of liver qi due to emotional frustration and stress is called liver depression qi stagnation in Chinese medicine.

Liver depression qi stagnation can result in a wide range of health problems including PMS, chronic digestive disturbance and depression. It can also play a role in rheumatic *bi* conditions. It is essential to keep the liver qi flowing as freely as possible. There are a number of effective ways to maintain a free flow of liver qi which will be explored later in this book.

2. The liver is said to store the blood. This means that, when the body is at rest, the blood in the extremities returns to the liver. It is said in Chinese medicine that the liver is yin in form but yang in function. Thus the liver requires sufficient blood to keep it and its associated tissues moist and supple, cool and relaxed.

3. The liver is said to control the sinews. The sinews here refer to the tendons and ligaments in the body. The proper functioning of the tendons and ligaments depends upon the nourishment of 'liver blood' to keep them moist and supple. Chronic rheumatic *bi* problems often involve the tendons and ligaments that surround the joints. Thus the connection between the tendons

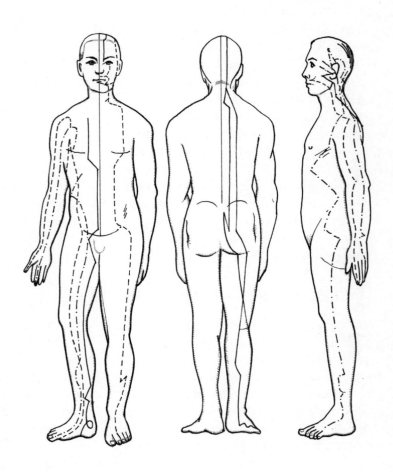

and ligaments and the liver's function of spreading the qi have implications for the treatment of chronic rheumatic *bi* pain. As we will see below, in all *chronic* rheumatic *bi* conditions, both the liver and the kidneys are believed to be lacking or deficient and need to be supplemented.

The relationship between the liver and rheumatic *bi* complaints is explained by two of the above statements. First, the liver controls the smooth flow of qi throughout the body. If the liver is unable to maintain this free flow of qi there will be problems of stagnation and possibly blockage. Secondly, the liver has a close relationship with the blood. If the blood is insufficient, the sinews will become dry and unable to relax. In Chinese medicine blood has a close relationship with essence. It is said, 'The blood and essence share a common source', and 'the liver and kidneys share a common source'. This means that blood insufficiency may lead to essence insufficiency and vice versa. It also means that liver disease eventually damages the kidneys. Thus many chronic conditions including chronic rheumatic *bi* problems involve both the liver and kidneys.

THE CHANNELS AND NETWORK VESSELS

Each viscus and bowel has a corresponding channel or meridian with which it is connected. In Chinese medicine, the inside of the body is made up of the viscera and bowels. The outside of the body is composed of the sinews and bones, muscles and flesh, and skin and hair. It is the channels and network vessels which connect the inside and the outside of the body. It is through these channels and network vessels that the viscera and bowels connect with their corresponding body tissues.

This channel and network vessel system is a unique feature of Chinese medicine. These channels and vessels are different from the circulatory, nervous or lymph systems. The earliest reference to them is in The *Nei Jing (The Inner Classic)*, a text written around the 2nd or 3rd century BCE.

The channels and vessels perform two basic functions. They are the pathways by which the qi and blood circulate through the body and between the organs and tissues. Additionally, the channels connect the internal organs with the exterior part of the body. This channel and vessel system functions in the body much like a communication network. The channels allow the various parts of our body to cooperate and interact to maintain our lives.

The channel and network vessel system is complex. There are 12 so-called regular channels, six yin and six yang, each with a specific pathway through the external body and connecting with an internal organ (see diagram page 25). There are also extraordinary vessels, channel sinews, channel divergences, main network vessels, and ultimately countless finer and finer network vessels permeating the entire body. All of these form a circuit that is similar to, but energetically distinct from, the circulatory system of Western medicine.

SUMMARY

It is my hope that this chapter has given you an appreciation for and a basic understanding of some of the fundamentals of Chinese medicine. In Chinese medicine, nothing stands alone. Every part and function in the body *co-responds* to other bodily parts and functions. The body, mind and spirit form an integrated whole. Health is the harmonious interaction of all the various aspects that comprise the organism. Disease and pain result when there is a disruption to this fundamental harmony and balance. In Chinese medicine, the focus of treatment is the restoration of harmony. Next, we will look at the cause of pain and explore rheumatic *bi* conditions according to Chinese medical thought.

PAIN ACCORDING
TO CHINESE MEDICINE

As was previously discussed, rheumatic complaints in Chinese medicine are classified as *bi*, and, whenever there is *bi* or impediment, there is pain. The following simple yet profound statement sums up the very essence of the Chinese medical view of pain:

If there is free flow, there is no pain;
If there is no free flow, there is pain.

This means that, as long as qi and blood flow freely and smoothly without hindrance or obstruction there is no pain in the body. However, if, *for any reason*, the flow of qi and blood is hindered, blocked, obstructed or does not flow freely, then there will be pain. Thus, in Chinese medicine, pain is simply the felt experience of lack of free flow of the qi and blood. As an extension of this, all joint pain is simply the experience of the lack of free flow of the qi and blood.

There are two main causes of the lack of free flow of the qi and blood. Either 1) something is hindering, blocking or obstructing the smooth and uninhibited flow of qi and blood through the channels and vessels, or 2) there is insufficient qi and blood to maintain smooth and free flow. In the first case, lack of free flow is like a blocked drain. The water cannot flow freely because something is physically obstructing the pipe. In the second case, either there is insufficient qi to push the blood or insufficient blood to maintain uninterrupted flow. Just as a stream dries up in late summer and is eventually reduced to pools of disconnected water, these pools just sit and no longer flow together. This is like the lack of free flow due to insufficient blood.

All pain, no matter what its Western medical diagnosis, is considered by Chinese medicine as a problem with the free flow of qi and blood. The Chinese medicine practitioner's job is first to diagnose the reason for the non-free flow of qi and blood and, second, to provide treatment to help restore it.

The flow of qi and blood can become inhibited in any and every area of the body: the internal organs, the muscles, the head, the low back, and the extremities and joints. For example, when we overeat and have acute indigestion with the accompanying feelings of abdominal fullness, bloating and distention, these symptoms are due to the stagnation of stomach qi. The stomach qi cannot move freely through the excessive amount of food and drink in the stomach. Likewise, when we bruise ourselves and blood escapes from the blood vessels and then pools, we experience a mild form of blood stagnation, technically called blood stasis in Chinese medicine. In both these cases, the stagnation is not serious. We are soon recovered and free of symptoms when the qi and blood resume their proper functioning and flow freely.

According to Chinese medicine, the sensations of pain due to qi stagnation or blood stasis are different. Qi stagnation causes a feeling of distention or soreness that fluctuates in intensity and location. Qi stagnation pain often occurs with strong emotional changes. Blood stasis, on the other hand, is characterised by painful swelling or stabbing sharp pain at a specific, fixed location.

It is also possible for the qi and blood flow to become inhibited because of insufficiency of the qi, blood or both. If this is the case, the pain is not severe but is enduring. If it is due to qi and blood insufficiency, the pain is worse after rest and better after light use. This is because, during rest or immobilisation, there is insufficient qi and blood to keep the qi and blood moving. Movement itself helps to pump the qi and blood through the mobilised area. Therefore, movement tends to make this type of pain better.

If the pain is primarily due to qi insufficiency, it will become worse by the end of the day or after excessive exercise. This is because the activity or exercise has used up the qi and left it even more deficient. Blood insufficiency pain tends to be worse at night after the scarce supply of blood has been consumed by the activities of the day and when it returns to the liver for storage.

In order for a Chinese medical practitioner to diagnose and treat rheumatic *bi* conditions, the following questions must be answered:

1. Is the pain due to blockage of the qi and blood or is it due more to the insufficiency of qi and blood?
2. If the pain is due to blockage, is the pain more characteristic of qi stagnation or blood stasis?
3. What are the factors or pathogens that are causing the qi and blood stagnation?
4. Which channels or network vessels are primarily involved in the pain?
5. Which internal organs are involved?

The answers to these questions will determine the treatment the patient receives from their Chinese medical practitioner. The basic principle of treatment in Chinese medicine is to restore balance. Therefore, The *Nei Jing (The Inner Classic)* says that, if a disease is due to an excess, then the correct treatment is to drain. If it is due to a deficiency, then the correct treatment is to supplement. If it is due to heat, the heat should be cooled. If it is due to cold, the cold should be warmed. If it is due to dryness, the dryness should be moistened. Finally, if it is due to dampness, the dampness should be dried.

In Chinese medicine, two patients with the same Western medical disease may receive quite different Chinese medical treatment because the root cause of their disease is not the same. Every patient in Chinese medicine is given individual treatment based on the cause and nature of their particular pattern of disharmony.

THE FOUR BASIC TYPES OF BI CONDITIONS

In the previous chapter, we saw that all pain is a reflection of a lack of free flow of either or both the qi and blood. We also saw that qi and blood may not flow freely because they either are blocked for some reason or there simply is not enough qi and blood to promote and maintain their flow. In Chinese medicine, rheumatic *bi* which is not associated with a known traumatic injury is typically ascribed to blockage by either wind, cold, dampness or heat. These are the four basic types of *bi* conditions in Chinese medicine. In such cases, any one or a combination of two or more of these pathological energies may be lodged in the channels and network vessels where they are not supposed to be. The result is that the qi and blood which should be freely and smoothly flowing through the channels and vessels will be blocked. Such pathological wind, cold, dampness or heat may either invade the body from outside or, and especially in the case of dampness and heat, may be produced internally due to a number of possible factors.

EXTERNAL ENVIRONMENTAL PATHOGENS

In Chinese medicine, there are three broad categories of disease causes. These categories are external causes, internal causes and a category which is neither internal nor external causes. The external causes of disease are called external environmental excesses. There are six of these external environmental excesses or pathogens. They are wind, cold, dampness, heat, dryness and summer heat. Any of these six factors may invade the body if either of two conditions exist. First, if one or more of these factors is unusually strong or unseasonable. For example, very cold weather in the middle of summer or very warm weather in the middle of winter may allow these 'excesses' to breach the body's defensive qi and invade. Secondly, if a person's defensive qi is weaker than it should be, any of these external pathogens if present in the environment may 'take advantage of this vacuity, and enter'. The *Nei Jing (The Inner Classic)* says, 'If evils enter, there must be vacuity.' This implies that evils can enter only if the defensive qi is weaker than it should be. However, there are times when the pathogenic qi in the external environment is so strong and virulent that it can breach the stoutest defence. This is known as epidemic or pestilential qi.

INTERNALLY ENGENDERED PATHOGENS

Although wind, cold, dampness and heat may all potentially invade the body from outside, three of these, cold, dampness and heat may also be produced internally. If, for any reason, there is insufficient yang qi, the body will not be as warm as it should be. The absence of heat will lead to cold. Yang qi may be damaged by overexposure to a cold environment, in which case the body exhausts itself in simply maintaining body temperature. Yang qi may be damaged by overeating uncooked, chilled foods and drinking chilled liquids, because in the process of digestion everything that goes into the stomach is turned into 100°F soup. Yang qi may be damaged and depleted by any loss of yin fluids, since yin fluids are the foundation or root of yang qi. Such loss of yin fluids includes bleeding, massive sweating and continual vomiting, diarrhoea or urination. Yang qi also becomes insufficient due to the decline of visceral function due to the ageing process. If the yang qi is insufficient to warm the body properly, it will not propel the blood and body fluids as it should. Instead, there is constriction and blockage of flow or *bi*.

Dampness may also be created internally. If the spleen is damaged and becomes weak or vacuous it will no longer move bodily fluids properly. Fluids will gather and collect and transform into dampness. Too much worrying or obsessive thinking, overeating sweets or other damp-producing foods such as dairy produce, wheat flour, fruit juices, oils and fats, or too little exercise may also damage the spleen. Dampness is a yin substance and it impedes the free flow of yang qi, thus resulting in *bi*. In addition, it is said in The *Nei Jing (The Inner Classic)* that the spleen declines at around 35 years of age. So, the spleen naturally weakens as a person ages. Consequently, one's ability to move and transform body fluids is not as good the older one gets past a certain age.

Heat may also be engendered internally. It does not have to invade from outside. In fact, in terms of rheumatic *bi* conditions, it does so relatively rarely. In order to understand how pathological heat is engendered internally resulting in *bi*, one must understand that the body's healthy or correct qi (also called the righteous qi) is inherently warm in nature. If this qi backs up and accumulates for any reason, then it will manifest as heat. This is called transformative or depressive heat. It may be due to liver depression qi stagnation in turn transforming into depressive heat or it may be due to any other cause of blockage and obstruction. For instance, if dampness, blood, food or phlegm gather and obstruct the free flow of yang qi, this may cause the accumulation of depressive or transformative heat. In real terms this means that even if one has sufficient righteous qi , if there is an enduring or severe accumulation, then damp *bi* or even cold *bi* may transform into heat *bi*.

WIND

Wind is usually the primary environmental factor to invade the body. In Chinese medicine it is known as the spearhead of disease. Wind in this instance does not necessarily mean windy weather. It refers to an unseen pathogen which affects the body and provokes a series of responses characteristic or reminiscent of the nature of environmental wind. Thus, a person with a windy type of pain will feel discomfort that comes and goes and moves around the body from joint to joint. Just as wind moves about the earth, the person's complaints shift throughout the body. As wind *bi*'s nature is changeable or movable, this type of impediment is called movable *bi*. In reality, wind as an external environmental pathogen typically combines with one of the other three. In Chinese medicine, the wind of wind *bi* is primarily seen as due to external invasion.

COLD

The emblem of cold in the natural world is ice, and, therefore, when cold causes *bi* or impediment, its nature and symptoms are reminiscent of ice. The pain of cold *bi* is worsened by exposure to cold and improved by warmth or heat. As cold is so constricting to the flow of liquids, the pain tends to be quite intense. So, cold *bi* is also called painful *bi*. Just as water becomes immobile when it turns to ice, so cold *bi* also tends to be fixed in location. Cold-producing *bi* may be due to either external invasion or internal production. If someone is said to be suffering from cold *bi*, this means the nature of their complaints share the characteristics of cold.

DAMPNESS

Dampness is an accumulation of water or body fluids in the body. Because dampness is like a flood, the affected area is typically swollen and oedematous. As water tends to run downwards, dampness tends to affect the lower part of the body more often than the upper part. As water is heavy, damp *bi* tends to be stationary. It does not move around from joint to joint. It is worsened by exposure to dampness and may be improved when the weather or surroundings are clear and dry. In addition, dampness tends to be lingering. Typically, damp *bi* has a slow and insidious onset and then a long drawn-out course. Its pain is most often dull but persistent. Like cold, which was discussed above, *bi* caused by dampness may be due to invasion either by external dampness or by internally created dampness. Both are common in the UK which has rather a damp climate.

HEAT

Redness is the colour which corresponds to fire or heat in Chinese medicine. Therefore if there is heat *bi* the affected area is typically red. Heat *bi* or impediment is rarely due to external invasion of hot pathogens. It is most commonly a result of an acute exacerbation of other types of *bi.*

QI STAGNATION, BLOOD STASIS AND PHLEGM NODULATION

Most cases of rheumatic *bi* or impediment involve the pathogens of wind, cold, dampness and/or heat. This is why, in Chinese, the word rheumatic is translated as *feng shi*, wind dampness. Regardless of whether these impediments are externally invading or internally created, they are often complicated by other factors involving the free flow of the qi and blood. Three of these factors are qi stagnation, blood stasis, and phlegm nodulation.

QI STAGNATION

Qi stagnation is often a result of emotional upset, stress and frustration. These factors affect the liver's ability to function properly. The resulting stagnation will affect the flow of qi and blood throughout the entire body and could lead to damp accumulation, phlegm obstruction, and/or food stagnation. In terms of joint pain, we already know that, 'If there is pain, there is no free flow', and in the preceding chapter we have taken a look at the four main types of rheumatic *bi* conditions. It is highly likely that liver depression qi stagnation will complicate and aggravate most if not all rheumatic *bi* complaints. The accumulation of dampness or heat in the body leading to impediment and pain may be directly caused by qi stagnation. Alternatively if there is an impediment or pain resulting from one of the pathogenic factors, it will produce qi stagnation.

BLOOD STASIS

Static blood, also known as dead blood, malign blood, vanquished blood and dry blood, means blood that is not moving. It obstructs the free flow of the channels and vessels in the same way as silt obstructs the flow of a river or stream. Static blood may be the result of traumatic injury. If the traumatic injury severs the channels and vessels, the blood moves outside its vessels and then pools and accumulates. The blood can only keep flowing as long as it is inside its vessels. Once there is the condition of static blood, this yin accumulation then impedes the flow of qi and body fluids. This is why traumatic injuries are followed by swelling and inflammation. The vessels are severed and blood flows outside them. The flow of qi and body fluids is impeded, body fluids gather and accumulate and result in oedema. Qi, which is yang, accumulates and results in heat and redness or inflammation. Later, when the vessels are repaired, the qi moves the blood and body fluids through the vessels. The swelling goes down, the redness and heat disappears, but the static blood which is left behind manifests as a 'black and blue mark'.

Because of the reciprocal relationship between the qi and blood, long-term qi stagnation will lead to blood stasis. As it is said in Chinese, 'If the qi moves, the blood moves; if the qi stops, the blood stops.' Therefore, anything that hinders and impedes the flow of qi will tend eventually to cause the complication of blood stasis. This could be due to emotional upset and frustration. Externally invading or internally engendered *bi* will also, over time, tend to become complicated by blood stasis. As the blood and body fluids flow together, if one of these gathers and collects, it will obstruct the free flow of the other. This means that dampness (or phlegm transformed out of dampness) over time will tend to become complicated by blood stasis, while long-term blood stasis will tend to become complicated by dampness and/or phlegm.

PHLEGM NODULATION

According to Chinese medical theory, phlegm results from accumulated dampness which has congealed into a thicker, denser form. Dampness may transform into phlegm if dampness simply endures for a long time. It may also congeal into phlegm due to either cold or heat. In the case of cold, it congeals dampness into phlegm like cold congeals water into ice. In the case of heat, it congeals dampness into phlegm like cooking something on a stove, the heat causing the fluids to thicken and condense. Once phlegm is produced, it obstructs and hinders the free flow of the qi, blood and healthy body fluids. Such phlegm is typically produced by the internal organs, and especially the spleen which is in charge of moving and transforming body fluids. Once produced, it often accumulates in the channels and vessels or in the space between the 'muscles and flesh' and the 'skin and hair'. If it accumulates in either the channels and vessels or in the space between the muscles and skin, it may form into phlegm nodules, lumps of non-moving, rubbery 'phlegm'. The nodulations associated with chronic, advanced rheumatic conditions are commonly considered, at least in part, phlegm nodulations in Chinese medicine.

JOINT CONTRACTURE AND DEFORMATION

If *bi* or impediment persists in an area, it will prevent the local tissue from obtaining its proper nourishment. If sinews fail to obtain proper nourishment, especially blood, they will wither, dry out and contract. The sinews in Chinese medicine refer to the tendons, ligaments and other connective tissues so contracture of the sinews due to localised malnourishment may lead to an inability to flex and extend the affected joint(s). In the same way enduring *bi* or impediment may prevent the bones from obtaining their proper nourishment. The bones may become deformed. This process of deformation is accelerated or worsened if there is lingering heat impediment, which is very damaging to the bones.

QI AND BLOOD VACUITY

In Chinese medicine, it is believed that the spleen begins to decline some time in one's mid-30s due to ageing. The spleen in Chinese medicine is the main viscus in charge of the production of qi and blood transformed from the food and drink we ingest. If there is insufficient qi and blood, it may result in joint pain for two basic reasons. First, the defensive qi that protects the exterior of the body from invasion by the six environmental excesses is produced from the digestate. If there is spleen weakness and vacuity, there may also be a resulting deficiency of this defensive qi. This would lead to the person being more easily invaded by the six environmental excesses. We have seen that four of these may cause *bi* within the body: wind, cold, dampness and heat. Secondly, if there is a spleen qi vacuity, there may not be sufficient qi to ensure the movement of the blood and body fluids, while there may not be enough blood to nourish and maintain healthy, working sinews and vessels. Therefore, a lack of sufficient qi and blood may lead to a lack of free flow, not because of *bi* per se, but because there is not enough qi and blood to keep the qi and blood flowing freely.

Chinese medicine, recognises that sometimes joint pain is not due to *bi*. Sometimes joint pain is simply due to a lack of sufficient qi and blood to keep the joints healthy and the qi and blood flowing freely. This scenario is typically seen in older patients. Within Chinese medicine, there are disease categories called '40-year shoulder' and '50-year wrist'. In these instances, pain is typically worse after the person has been resting for some time. When we are at rest, our blood is stored in the liver and our qi is not mobilised to our extremities. Thus the sinews are less nourished and the qi and blood flow is not as free. When we try to use the joint after being at rest, at first it is sore and stiff.

However, the movement itself promotes the flow of qi and blood. As the qi and blood flow more and more to and through the joint, the soreness and stiffness disappear.

In cases where there is little or no actual _bi_ or impediment, but the soreness and stiffness is mainly due to insufficiency of qi and blood, then too much exercise or overexertion may worsen the situation. All activity involves consumption of qi and blood. Since activity consumes qi and blood in the same way as a car uses petrol, overconsumption will lead to a worsening of any symptoms associated with insufficiency of the qi and blood. While light exercise or mobilisation relieves soreness and stiffness due to qi and blood insufficiency, heavy exercise or overexertion may make the situation worse. Since qi and blood are consumed by daily life, such symptoms are often worse in the evening or at night after we have been consuming qi and blood all day.

SPLEEN VACUITY

Factors which may lead to spleen vacuity or deficiency are overexertion, excessive blood loss, worrying and obsessive thinking or an incorrect diet. Since the spleen plays a pivotal role in the production of qi and blood, consumption of too much qi and/or blood loss can exhaust the spleen. As women lose blood on a monthly basis during menstruation they are more prone to spleen vacuity than men. This offers some explanation as to why women, particularly younger women, tend to have more systemic rheumatic complaints than men of the same age.

While too much thinking, especially worry and anxiety, can damage the spleen, an incorrect diet is a main cause of spleen vacuity, particularly in the West. Overeating uncooked, chilled foods damages the spleen, as does overeating sugars and sweets and damp, phlegm-producing foods. According to Chinese medicine, such damp-engendering, phlegm-producing foods include the following:

Milk	Wheat flour products
Cheese	Most fruits and fruit juices
Yoghurt	Tomatoes
Oils and fats	Most nuts

If a person's spleen is vacuous and weak to begin with, these 'heavy', harder to digest foods will overwhelm the spleen and damage it. They will tend to create or aggravate the presence of pathological dampness and phlegm. It is said in Chinese, 'The spleen is averse to dampness.' Therefore, diet is an important factor if joint pain is associated with either qi and blood vacuity or the presence of dampness and phlegm. This includes a number of rheumatic diseases, including RA and systemic lupus erythematosus (SLE).

KIDNEY VACUITY

The low back or lumbar region is said to be the 'mansion' of the kidneys. The bones and joints are governed by the kidneys. Kidney vacuity or weakness is often associated with low back soreness and pain and may be associated with spinal column pain and deformation. As the kidneys begin to become weak after 40 years of age due to the ageing process, this contributes to an increase of bone and joint problems. In general, most people who have systemic diseases, such as RA and SLE, which involve rheumatic pain, according to Chinese medicine, have some element of spleen and/or kidney vacuity.

TREATMENT BASED ON PATTERN DISCRIMINATION

Chinese medical diagnosis is different from a patient's named disease or illness in Western terms. In Chinese medicine treatment is given based on an individual diagnosis rather than a named disease or illness. In Traditional Chinese Medicine, or TCM* as it is commonly known, groups of symptoms are put together to form a pattern. This pattern then becomes the basis for diagnosis and treatment. It is said according to Chinese medicine:

One disease, different treatments.
Different diseases, same treatment.

The result is that two patients may receive different Chinese medical treatments *if their Chinese patterns are different*, while two patients with different named diseases may receive the same treatment *if their Chinese patterns are the same*. A patient with rheumatic *bi* due to wind, cold and dampness with spleen yang vacuity, for example, will receive a completely different treatment from a patient with rheumatic *bi* with kidney yin vacuity. While both patients could have the identical Western medical diagnosis of rheumatoid arthritis, each would have totally different sign and symptom complexes from the Chinese medical point of view. This individual pattern diagnosis and treatment is beneficial in that it produces no side effects or medically induced problems.

A person's Chinese pattern takes into account the signs and symptoms of the disease or illness plus many other factors

---

* TCM is the main method of practising Chinese medicine which is widely used in both the West and modern China.

which may be seemingly unrelated to the illness. All the person's symptoms are of interest, not just those which relate to the main complaint. It is probably true to say that a practitioner of Chinese medicine will spend longer initially questioning the patient than his/her Western counterpart.

As we have seen in the previous chapters, rheumatic *bi* conditions are due to a lack of free flow of the qi and/or blood due to impediment by wind, cold, damp or heat as well as qi stagnation, blood stasis, phlegm nodulation, qi and blood vacuity, and vacuities of the spleen and kidneys. This means that there are a number of different factors accounting for any given person's individual rheumatic complaints. In Chinese medicine, each patient with a rheumatic complaint or joint pain will receive an individually tailored treatment plan based on their own specific pattern of disharmony. Only by taking account of *all* the person's signs and symptoms can the practitioner begin to identify the factors that contribute to the patient's rheumatic *bi* condition.

Vital to a Chinese medical diagnosis are what are known as: The four examinations. We will now look at these in greater depth.

THE FOUR EXAMINATIONS

These examinations or methods of diagnosis have been an integral part of Chinese medicine over the centuries. The four examinations are 1) looking, 2) listening/smelling, 3) asking, and 4) touching.

1. Looking, as one would expect, focuses on what the practitioner can see. Everything about a patient that can be observed can be useful. This includes their facial expression, the brightness of their eyes, skin tone and complexion, bodily constitution, posture and manner of movement, appearance of the affected area and of the tongue and its coating.

Tongue diagnosis is a highly developed skill in Chinese medicine and may be a major source of information about a patient's condition. For example, a thick, greasy, yellow tongue coating indicates the presence of damp heat, while a shiny, red tongue without a coating indicates a yin vacuity.

2. Listening and smelling are put in the same category of diagnosis. This is because the character in the Chinese language for this examination includes them both as a single concept. The practitioner listens to the patient's breathing, the quality of their voice, or other sounds, such as a cough. A person, for example, with a weak voice who coughs when active may have weak qi. The use of the sense of smell may at first seem surprising but when someone is out of balance or has an illness they sometimes have a certain body odour that gives further information with regard to their underlying imbalance.

3. Questioning the patient is another crucial part of the examination. These questions include when and how the problem happened, how long it has gone on, what treatment has already been given and with what results, general medical history, sensations of cold and heat, location and quality of pain, descriptions of urination and bowel movements, sleep patterns, perspiration, headaches, dizziness, appetite, thirst, digestive disturbances, energy level, gynaecological problems, and more. The patient's description of the pain may be critical in determining what type of *bi* or what type of pattern exists.

4. The final examination of the four is touch. By touching and palpating various areas of the body the practitioner can know and understand the condition of the body and its internal organs.

An important aspect of this method, at least in terms of assessing viscera, bowel function and basic quantities and qualities of qi and blood flow, is pulse diagnosis. Chinese pulse diagnosis requires skill and sensitivity. The pulse, which may be taken at the wrist, provides information about the basic state of the person's qi and blood, yin and yang, viscera and bowels, and pathogenic factors. There are 28 different standard pulse qualities described in the classical medical literature. For example, people in pain who have a lot of qi and blood typically have a pulse which is tight 'like a taut rope', while people in pain with less qi and blood typically have a pulse which is wiry 'like the string of a zither'.

By gathering information through the four examinations and by comparing the patient's signs and symptoms with the condition of the tongue and pulse, the patient's pattern is diagnosed. The diagnosis itself describes an inherent state of imbalance. For example, kidney yin insufficiency means that kidney yin is too weak. The next step is to create a treatment plan that will correct the imbalance. If there is kidney yin vacuity, the kidneys should be supplemented and yin should be nourished or enriched. Treatment is given to bring about this result, thus return to balance and, therefore, health.

CHINESE TREATMENT METHODS FOR RHEUMATIC *BI*

Once a practitioner of Chinese medicine has determined an individual's pattern of disharmony, a treatment plan is formed. There are three main treatment methods which may be used. These are: acupuncture (including moxibustion), Chinese herbal medicine and Chinese or Oriental medical massage. These treatment methods may be used in combination with each other as we will see in a later chapter.

ACUPUNCTURE

What is acupuncture?

cupuncture primarily means the insertion of extremely thin, sterilised, stainless steel needles into specific points on the body where there are special concentrations of qi and blood. Therefore, these points have a special regulatory influence and balance the flow of qi and blood over the channel and network system we described above. As we have seen above, the pain experienced as an integral part of rheumatic *bi* complaints is due to a loss of free flow of the qi and blood. Since acupuncture seeks to regulate the flow of qi and blood directly and immediately through the channels and vessels, acupuncture is an especially good treatment option for eliminating *bi* pain. In China, acupuncture is so well known for its effective treatment of all sorts of bi conditions that the treatment of rheumatic complaints makes up a major part of most acupuncturists' practices.

As a generic term, acupuncture also includes several other methods of stimulating acupuncture points, thus regulating the flow of qi in the body. The other main modality is moxibustion. This means the warming of acupuncture points mainly by burning dried, aged Oriental mugwort on, near or over acupuncture points. The purposes of this warming treatment are to 1) stimulate the flow of qi and blood even more strongly, 2) add warmth to areas of the body that are too cold, and 3) add yang qi to the body to supplement a yang qi vacuity. Because the warmth of moxibustion is an immediate and specific remedy for cold *bi*, moxibustion is almost always used to treat that kind of impediment. However, because moxibustion does move the qi and quicken the blood more powerfully than acupuncture, it is also used to treat non-cold *bi* that is enduring or recalcitrant, *i.e.*, stubborn to treatment.

Other acupuncture modalities are to apply suction cups over points, to prick the points to allow a drop or two of blood to exit, to apply magnets to the points, to warm the points with various types of heat lamps, and to stimulate the points by either electricity or laser.

What is a typical acupuncture treatment like?
There are quite a few different styles or methods of working with acupuncture and some aspects of treatment will vary from practitioner to practitioner depending on their training. However, there are certain aspects which remain the same: all practitioners will take a case history and gather information so that they can make a diagnosis. They will also use various methods to make an Oriental medical diagnosis, will almost certainly take the pulse at the wrist and may examine the tongue and abdomen.

Once the diagnosis has been made, the treatment will begin and very fine stainless steel needles will be inserted into selected points on the body. It is unusual for more than 15 needles to be inserted during a treatment so you won't end up looking like a pin cushion! The needles used are generally disposable, but if not they are sterilised according to hospital safety standards. There is no need to be concerned about infection as a properly trained acupuncturist who is a member of the relevant professional body must comply with strict standards of safety. The needles may be manipulated gently after insertion and they may be left in for up to 30 minutes until the acupuncturist feels the desired effect has been achieved. Some practitioners may use an electro-acupuncture machine which is attached to the needles to stimulate the qi or energy flow further.

Moxibustion may also be used, either on the needles or directly on the skin. Whatever the technique it is normally a pleasant warm sensation and will not burn the patient.

Does acupuncture hurt?

In Chinese, it is said that acupuncture is *bu tong*, painless. However, patients may feel some mild soreness, heaviness, electrical tingling or distension. For most people the sensation is acceptable and not really painful, although needle techniques vary and people do have different pain thresholds.

Ear acupuncture

Some acupuncturists may also use points in the ear to treat arthritis. Needles may be used during the acupunture session to stimulate specific points on the ear. Alternatively tiny metal pellets, seeds or special press needles are used which are covered with adhesive plaster and may be left in for a few days to support the treatment. In this way the effectiveness and duration of treatment may be enhanced.

CHINESE HERBAL MEDICINE

Herbal medicine has been used in China for thousands of years, and the materia medica or repertoire of healing ingredients includes over 5,000 substances. Most often a remedy or formula is given which includes between three and twenty different herbs or medicinals. Over the centuries these herbal formulas have been tried and tested many times.

Herbs are now available in a number of formats, both traditional and modern. The traditional method is to make a tea or use pills. The herbs are now commonly available as freeze-dried powders or tinctures. The herbs will certainly taste unusual at first to someone who has not tried them before, but the vast majority of people get used to the taste quite quickly.

In modern China, herbal medicine is widely used for the treatment of arthritis. In the UK there are far fewer trained Chinese herbalists than acupuncturists, although some acupuncturists are trained in the use of traditional remedies known as 'patents'. There are many of these traditional 'patent' remedies that are very useful for treating arthritic and rheumatic conditions.

In the UK it is not possible to buy Chinese herbal medicines from a reputable supplier unless you have a prescription from a trained practitioner. We would strongly recommend that you seek professional advice from a fully qualified practitioner when taking Chinese herbs.

ORIENTAL MEDICAL MASSAGE

Medical massage in China is called *tui na*. It has developed into a high art and is practised extensively in hospitals where there is often a special ward or clinic within the hospital devoted to it. Like acupuncture it works on the meridian or channel system, and specific strokes or manipulations move and regulate the flow of qi. At present there are not many practitioners of *tui na* in the UK, although it is growing in popularity.

Another form of Oriental medical massage is Shiatsu, which originates from Japan. This is a deeply relaxing therapy and there are quite a number of practitioners working in the UK. Shiatsu is done with the patient/client wearing loose, comfortable clothing. Diagnosis is mainly through gently palpating the abdomen to detect underlying imbalances in the person's energy. The relevant meridians or channels are then worked on to release blockages and strengthen areas of deficiency or vacuity. It may be a highly beneficial treatment for arthritis.

CASE HISTORIES

O ne of the best ways to illustrate how Chinese medicine works is through the presentation of case histories. Seeing Chinese medicine in action will hopefully give you a greater understanding of how it works to treat arthritis. These case histories will also demonstrate the holistic nature of Chinese medicine, showing how the whole person is treated, not just their disease or illness. Often other signs and symptoms improve as well as the main complaint.

The case histories will be presented in terms of pattern diagnosis categories from Traditional Chinese Medicine or TCM, the style of Chinese medicine that I use in my clinic.

EARLY STAGE RHEUMATIC PAIN

Wind, damp, exterior pattern

Kurt, age 27, was camping in the mountains over the weekend and was caught in a spring rainstorm while hiking. The next day, he awoke with a headache, a bit of a chill and a slight fever, and his body 'felt really heavy and sore all over, especially in the joints'. When I inspected his tongue, it was a normal colour with normal, thin, white fur. When I felt his pulse, it was floating and bowstring. Kurt contracted a wind damp condition in the superficial aspect and muscles of his body. The headache, heaviness of his body, and sore joints are indicative of pain due to damp *bi*. When dampness blocks the free flow of qi, there is achy pain. Conditions with sudden onset typically indicate that wind is involved. 'Wind' is the vector that commonly carries the other five environmental excesses into the body. In this case, damp was, therefore, combined with wind. The chills, slight fever, normal tongue and fur, and the floating pulse all indicated that he had an 'exterior' condition. The floating pulse indicates that his qi is not flowing freely.

Kurt's treatment included both acupuncture and Chinese herbal medicine to release or resolve the exterior portion of his body and to dispel the invading pathogenic factors of wind, eliminate dampness and stop pain. Acupuncture consisted of needling *Fu Liu* (Ki 7) and *He Gu* (LI 4), *Feng Men* (Bl 12) and *Feng Chi* (GB 20), and *Kun Lun* (Bl 60). The first two points promote perspiration, thus relieving the exterior and kicking the wind back out of the body. The second two points are called 'wind' points. In particular, they treat pain in the upper back, head and neck due to external invasion of wind. The last point is a point which releases the entire back of the body. It may be used when an external pathogen has lodged in the most superficial layer of the body resulting in pain.

In terms of Chinese herbal medicine, I prescribed *Qiang Huo Sheng Shi Tang* (Notopterygium Overcome Dampness Decoction), a standard formula for wind damp *bi* due to exterior invasion. It consisted of Radix Et Rhizoma Notopterygii (*Qiang Huo*), Radix Angelicae Pubescentis (*Du Huo*), Radix Et Rhizoma Ligustici (*Gao Ben*), Radix Ledebouriellae Divaricatae (*Fang Feng*), Radix Ligustici Wallichii (*Chuan Xiong*), Fructus Viticis (*Man Jing Zi*) and mix-fried Radix Glycyrrhizae (*Gan Cao*). These medicinals were boiled in three cups of water down to 1½ cup of liquid. The dregs were removed and Kurt was instructed to drink ½ cup three times that day. The next day, Kurt called me to say that he was feeling much better. The fever and chills had disappeared, his body no longer felt heavy, and his joint pain was gone. At a follow-up meeting two weeks later, Kurt said that there had been no further complications.

Wind, damp, heat, exterior pattern

Alice, age 26, had felt bad for two days. She had back pain, fever, slight chills, an achy feeling in her body, and red, swollen knees that felt hot to the touch. Her tongue was slightly red at the tip and had slightly yellow tongue fur. Her pulse was floating, bowstring, and rapid. Alice had contracted a wind damp heat condition. Alice's recent onset of fever and chills indicated the presence of an external factor that was still in the superficial part of her body. The fever and red-hot knees indicated the presence of heat. The swollen knees indicated the presence of dampness. The body achiness and leg pain was due to blockage of qi by this external dampness impediment. The red-tipped tongue and yellow fur indicated pathogenic heat, while the floating pulse confirmed an exterior pattern, the bowstring pulse confirmed that the qi was not flowing freely, and the rapid pulse confirmed the presence of pathological heat.

Like Kurt, Alice received an acupuncture treatment and some Chinese herbs. Her acupuncture consisted of *He Gu* (LI 4) and *Wai Guan* (TB 5), *Du Bi* (St 35) and *Nei Xi Yan* (M-LE- 16a), and *Yang Ling Quan* (GB 34) and *Yin Ling Quan* (Sp 9). The first two points in this treatment clear heat and resolve the exterior. The second pair treat knee pain by freeing the flow locally. The last pair also treat the local flow of qi and additionally they clear heat and eliminate dampness from the body in general.

The herbal formula Alice received contained Cortex Phellodendri (*Huang Bai*), Semen Coicis Lachryma-jobi (*Yi Yi Ren*), Rhizoma Atractylodis (*Cang Zhu*), Radix Achyranthis Bidentatae (*Niu Xi*), Radix Stephaniae Tetrandrae (*Han Fang Ji*), Radix Gentianae Macrocephalae (*Qin Jiao*) and Fructus Chaenomelis Lagenariae (*Mu Gua*), medicinals which clear heat, dispel wind, eliminate dampness and eliminate impediment specifically from the lower limbs.

The next day, Alice reported that the acupuncture treatment had really helped reduce the knee pain almost immediately. The feverish feeling was gone, but the knees still felt a little hot to the touch and there was still a little bit of 'hot' pain in the knees. So, I repeated the same prescription and instructed Alice to take it for another two days to make sure she recuperated completely. By the end of that time, the pain and hot feelings were eliminated. On follow-up after two weeks, there had been no recurrence.

Both Alice's and Kurt's rheumatic pains were clearly acute conditions. Both were of sudden onset which is one indication of invasion by wind. The fever and chills they each experienced are also a primary indicator of a superficial invasion of the body by external pathogens. According to Chinese medicine, invasions by environmental excesses may frequently first attack the exterior part of the body, that is the skin and muscles.

Kurt and Alice both were wise to seek immediate treatment. Chinese medicine strongly advises that superficial illness, such as they both had, be quickly and properly resolved. If the environmental factors are not dispersed and eliminated through either proper treatment or the body's own healing mechanisms, they can lodge in the channels and become the cause of chronic rheumatic/arthritic conditions. Remember, the longer a pathogenic factor blocks the flow of the qi and blood through the body, the more difficult it is to eliminate. Therefore rheumatic *bi* conditions, like many of life's challenges and problems, are best resolved early before they become more troublesome.

We are not always able to cope with illness when it arises. Frequently illnesses and health problems do resolve themselves without intervention. The natural healing ability of the body is at work. Sometimes, however, illnesses progress and do not resolve themselves: they become chronic.

Let's now look at what happens when a rheumatic condition progresses beyond the initial stages as seen in the two cases. This means that the symptoms of superficial invasion, *i.e.*, fever and chills, will not be present although, in some cases, the person may have fever accompanying their rheumatic pain. This type of fever is due to heat that is being internally generated. The cases that follow could be classified as true rheumatic conditions or *bi* conditions in Chinese medicine. The environmental factors, wind, cold and damp or wind, heat and damp, are lodged in the channels traversing the joints or other areas of the body, blocking the flow of qi and blood and causing pain.

CHRONIC RHEUMATIC PAIN

Wind, cold, damp *bi*

Tom was in his early 50s and worked as an area consultant for a multilevel marketing company. When he arrived for his first appointment, he had difficulty walking due to the pain in his left knee. He also had pain in the right elbow and left shoulder. The pain was aggravated by changes in the weather, especially rain and cold. His joints felt cold to the touch and were stiff. The only times he felt 'normal' were when he soaked in a hot bath. These hot soaks would ease his pain for an hour or two.

Tom had been playing a ball game in a gentle rain four months previously. He had been 'chilled to the bone'. That evening, he developed some sniffles and continued to feel chilled. For the next few days, he had felt achy all over and then the pain 'just settled into my joints'. He had hoped it would go away, but it hadn't.

Tom's condition was due to wind, cold and damp. Whereas, in Kurt's and Alice's cases described above, the invasion of external environmental excesses were resolved without further complication, Tom had developed an early stage rheumatic *bi* condition.

The original sniffles, chill and achiness were symptoms of wind, cold, damp invasion. The continued joint pain indicated that the pathogenic factors wind, cold and dampness had now lodged in the channels. The joint stiffness that got worse with rain, indicated the presence of damp. Changes in the barometric pressures that accompany the arrival of a new weather front can worsen damp conditions. The pain relief he experienced by soaking in a hot bath as well as the sensation of cold in his joints indicated the presence of cold. From a Western medical perspective, Tom's condition could indicate early stage rheumatoid arthritis, osteoarthritis or bursitis.

Tom was treated by a combination of acupuncture, moxibustion and Chinese medicinals. The focus of treatment was to dispel the wind, scatter the cold, eliminate the dampness and circulate the qi and blood through the channels traversing his painful joints. Points were needled around each joint as well as points on the channels along which the pain was felt. While the needles were in place, moxa (Folium Artemisiae Argyii, *Ai Ye*) was attached to and burned on the heads of the needles surrounding the affected joints. This is called warm needle technique. Tom received three treatments the first week, two treatments each the second and third weeks, and one treatment during week four. During this entire course of acupuncture treatment, he also took the Chinese herbal patent medicine, *Guan Jie Yan Wan* (Close Down Joint Inflammation Pills), eight pills each time, three times per day. These pills treat joint pain due to wind, damp, cold *bi*. Tom was given some Chinese medicinal plasters to apply externally to the most painful joints. These were called *Shang Shi Zhi Tong Gao* (Damage by Dampness, Stop Pain Plasters). Tom's pain was completely eliminated within one month following treatment with Chinese medicine.

Tom's condition was an early stage rheumatic wind, damp, cold *bi*. He had no symptoms or signs of weakness in any of his internal organs. The treatment focused upon removing the pathogens lodged in the channels traversing his painful joints. It is important to keep in mind that patients with a long-standing rheumatic *bi* condition will often show symptoms of spleen vacuity and/or dampness, liver depression and/or vacuity, and kidney yin and/or yang vacuity weakness. In cases such as these, the imbalance within the internal organ(s) must be addressed if the condition is to resolve. The focus of treatment in these cases needs to involve treating the affected organ(s) as well as removing the impeding factors that are blocking the free flow of qi and blood. We will now look at a number of cases that demonstrate the importance of treating the internal organs whilst at the same time addressing the rheumatic joint pain.

Chronic wind, cold, damp *bi* with a predominance of wind

Phyllis, 57, loved to run and hike. However, for the past three years, she'd dramatically reduced her activities due to pain in her elbows, knees and neck. Her Western doctor had diagnosed osteoarthritis and suggested she take NSAIDs (non-steroidal anti-inflammatory drugs) to control the pain. During Phyllis's Chinese medical exam, she said her pain had a tendency to move from joint to joint and varied from a sharp to a dull, achy sensation. 'Some days my knees hurt; other days it's my neck or my elbows.' She reported occasional numbness in the muscles of her forearms. Her pains tended to worsen under strong wind conditions which occurred frequently. Phyllis's low back was also achy and sore. She liked warmth and felt 'a bit better' when the weather was warm. Phyllis loved where she lived so that moving to a warmer, less windy climate was not a consideration.

Phyllis's Chinese medical diagnosis was wind, cold, damp *bi* with a predominance of wind, along with kidney vacuity. Two of Phyllis's symptoms were indicative of pain due to wind. When pain moves from joint to joint as it did in Phyllis's case, it is considered to be like the wind moving. Pains that change in quality, that are sometimes dull and sometimes sharp, are also indicative of pathogenic wind. The presence of cold was indicated by the fact that Phyllis deliberately sought warmth and found it effective in reducing her pain. Her low back pain was a sign that her kidneys were weak. This was corroborated by the fact that she got up twice to urinate each night, that her feet were particularly cold and that her libido was almost non-existent. Her age also suggested kidney vacuity as the kidney energies are typically weakened by or after the late 40s in women. The numbness in her forearm was due to the blockage of the qi and blood. It is said in The *Nei Jing* (*The Inner Classic*) that tissues can function and feel when they obtain blood to nourish them. If tissues are not properly nourished then numbness, or a lack of sensitivity, may occur.

Phyllis also received acupuncture, moxibustion and Chinese herbal medicine to dispel wind, scatter cold and eliminate dampness. Her treatment involved strengthening her kidneys and, in particular, kidney yang. In her case, the predominant pathogenic factor was wind, and this was combined with kidney vacuity weakness. Acupuncture and moxibustion (warm needle technique) was used to eliminate the pathogenic factors, while Chinese medicinals were used to strengthen the kidneys and the liver. Phyllis was prescribed the Chinese patent medicine, *Du Zhong Feng Shi Wan* (Eucommia Wind Damp Pills), four pills each time, twice a day. These pills include ingredients which dispel wind, scatter cold and eliminate dampness; they also supplement the kidneys and invigorate yang.

The kidneys are the foundation of the yin and yang. It is said that, 'enduring disease (eventually) reaches the kidneys'. When the kidneys are weak, the liver is also often weakened, especially in post-menopausal women. In Phyllis's case, there were no signs of liver weakness. A Chinese medical practitioner, however, always keeps in mind that the liver and kidneys 'share a common source'. In addition, the liver is responsible for nourishing the sinews, *i.e.*, ligaments and tendons, that are important tissues in all joints. The liver is also involved in ensuring that the qi flows smoothly through the body. With regard to all joint problems, it is important that the kidneys and the liver are healthy and functioning properly.

In Phyllis's case, we see two important principles in the treatment of rheumatic *bi* conditions according to Chinese medicine. First, we must determine what pathogenic factors are involved and in what proportion. In Phyllis's case, pathogenic wind was the most prominent pathogen. Having this knowledge enables the practitioner to tailor treatment primarily to dispel wind. There are specific acupuncture points and medicinals that dispel wind, just as there are acupuncture points and medicinals to scatter cold, eliminate dampness or clear heat. Second, it is essential to determine the strength of the internal organs. If the internal organs are weak, as is often the case in chronic conditions, it will be difficult, if not impossible, for treatment to be successful. In Phyllis's case, her kidneys needed to be strengthened to ensure recovery.

Wind, cold, damp _bi_ with a preponderance of cold

Ralph, 59, needed to take early retirement from his job as a plumber following a diagnosis of osteoarthritis. He had intense, sharp pains in his neck, shoulders and hands with a decrease in range of motion. He hated the cold because it made his pain worse. His painful joints were cold to the touch and so was his abdomen. Ralph also tended to have loose stools.

Ralph, like Phyllis above, had a wind, damp, cold _bi_ condition. However, the major pathogen in Ralph's case was cold. Pain due to cold is intense, sharp or even stabbing. This is because cold blocks the flow of qi and blood in the same way that cold freezes water into ice. When cold is the predominant pathogenic factor in an impediment condition, the person does not tolerate cold weather well. Cold weather 'adds' to the existing cold in the channels, causing even more stagnation of qi and blood and increasing the already intense pain. Ralph's tendency towards loose stools and abdominal coldness indicated that his spleen, specifically his spleen yang, was weak. Loose stools, especially after meals, and/or stools which contain undigested food, are major symptoms of spleen vacuity. Should someone have loose stools, a feeling of coldness, and the abdomen feels cold to the touch, these are certain signs that the warming aspect of the spleen, its yang aspect, is weak.

Cold rheumatic _bi_ conditions are treated by using warmth to scatter cold and warm yang. Ralph's treatment consisted of acupuncture, moxibustion and Chinese herbal medicinals to warm the channels, scatter cold and warmly supplement spleen yang. Moxibustion is an essential component in the treatment of pathogenic cold in the channels and helps to warm and fortify spleen yang. Ralph was given a moxibustion stick for home use so he could give himself daily treatments. He was prescribed *Xiao Huo Luo Dan* (Small Quicken the Network Vessels Elixir), a Chinese medicine which primarily treats cold *bi*. This was accompanied by another Chinese patent medicine, *Xiang Sha Liu Jun Zi Tang* (Auklandia and Amomum Six Gentlemen Pills), one of the most well-known Chinese formula for spleen vacuity loose stools.

Within only two days of beginning treatment, Ralph began to feel better. His joints began to feel warmer and the pain was considerably reduced. Ralph was advised to eat cooked foods and refrain from eating uncooked vegetables and fruits and chilled, iced or frozen foods and drinks, as these foods and beverages only add cold to cold and easily damage spleen yang. In Ralph's case, we wanted to protect and warm his spleen yang to disperse the cold that had accumulated in his neck, shoulders and arms.

Two cases of painful swollen red knees

The next two cases demonstrate how important it is in Chinese medicine to see rheumatic conditions holistically. At first glance, both individuals appear to have the same problem. Both have a red, painful, swollen knee. We shall see, however, that the causes were different, and, therefore, the treatments for these two patients were also quite different. If the same Chinese medical treatment were administered to both individuals, one of them would recover, while one could get much worse.

Craig was in his early 40s and worked as a computer programmer. He loved his work because he did not need to interact with many people. He felt that he was a very irritable person. For the past two years, his right knee was very painful. 'It will blow up like a balloon and get really red and hot. Most of the time, it's just a little swollen and red.' He'd tried a number of medications for his knee that helped for a short while but did not completely get rid of the pain. He came to see me to see if a more holistic approach to his problem might help.

Craig loved to put ice on his knee and, in fact, felt best when he soaked in a cold bath, even in winter. He hated summer because the heat was just too much. He drank ice water 'by the gallon' daily even in the winter and had a red face. He tended towards being constipated.

Craig has a classic case of damp heat *bi*. The swollen knee is a sign of pathogenic dampness. Signs of heat included irritability (*i.e.*, heat affecting the Chinese medical idea of the liver), redness in the knee and face (red is the colour of heat in Chinese medicine), thirst for cold beverages (heat damages and consumes body fluids and may cause a desire for cold drinks), and constipation (if the intestines are dried out by pathogenic heat, the stools will be too dry to move). In Craig's case, the heat was due to internal causes. There were no signs or symptoms such as fever and chill to indicate that he had had an external invasion. In addition, there was no history of the condition being initiated by an external pattern. His preference for cold, the use of ice on the knee, the cold soaks and a love of winter are all further evidence that Craig is systemically too hot.

Craig was treated by a combination of acupuncture and Chinese herbal medicine. He was prescribed the same formula as Alice above. However, to this formula, Radix Et Rhizoma Rhei (*Da Huang*) and Mirabilitum (*Mang Xiao*) were added to purge the bowels and clear heat specifically from the large intestine (and therefore also from the liver, according to Chinese medical theory). This formula relieved Craig's constipation at the same time as it reduced the pain and inflammation in his knee. Craig needed to be treated for two months before his knee pain went away entirely. To this day, if Craig overeats hot, peppery, greasy, oily, spicy foods and drinks too much alcohol, twinges of pain and his constipation return. In that case, he knows immediately to change to what Chinese medicine calls a 'clear, bland diet' and to purge his bowels with Milk of Magnesia. He has not had to receive any further acupuncture for several years.

Jan was also in her early 40s. She was a school teacher who loved her work. However, for the past year, her right knee had been bothering her more and more. She'd had pain in her knee for many years following a skiing injury. Initially, her knee had been swollen without redness. For the past few months, the knee had been swollen, red and hot, especially after a long week on her feet. Jan was easily chilled and loved warmth. 'It can never be too warm for me.' The thought of putting ice on her knee was not appealing even though it was hot to the touch. She tended to have swelling in her feet (oedema) along with loose stools and occasional low back pain.

Jan's knee pain was due to long-standing wind, cold and damp *bi* transforming into a wind, damp, heat *bi* condition. Over time and given the right bodily constitution and conditions, some patient's wind, cold, damp rheumatic *bi* will transform into a heat *bi* condition. Her original cold, damp knee problem was now a localised damp heat problem. Unlike Craig above, Jan's swollen, red-hot knees were the only heat signs and symptoms she had. Everything else pointed to a cold and damp condition. Her love of warmth and dislike of cold and her loose stools indicated vacuity cold due to a weakness of her spleen yang. The swelling of the knee and the oedema in the feet were signs of excessive dampness in her body. In fact, Jan's cold, damp constitutional condition was due to a weakness of her kidney and spleen yang, the oedema being due to both the spleen and kidneys being too weak to move and transform body fluids properly, while the low back pain was a classic kidney vacuity symptom in a woman her age.

For her treatment, Jan received the same herbal formula as Alice and Craig. Unlike Craig, however, Radix Et Rhizoma Rhei and Mirabilitum were not added. Instead, this formula was combined with the Chinese patent medicine *Shen Ling Bai Zhu Pian* (Ginseng, Poria and Atractylodes Tablets), a well-known formula for treating spleen vacuity. Acupuncture was used locally in order to drain off the depressed qi (*i.e.*, heat) and move the dampness. Moxibustion was applied to the points on the back that supplement the spleen and kidneys (*Pi Shu*, Bl 20, and *Shen Shu*, Bl 23, respectively). In addition, moxibustion was also performed at *Guan Yuan* (CV 4) and *Zhong Wan* (CV 12), one on the lower abdomen and the other on the upper abdomen, in order to also help supplement and warm the kidneys and spleen. After a total of eight acupuncture treatments, her red, swollen, painful knees were much improved. The herbal formula in decoction was discontinued as was the insertion of needles around the knees. Jan's husband was taught how to do the moxibustion on her back and abdomen in order to continue supplementing the kidneys and spleen for two months further. She continued to take the Chinese pills until her stools were no longer loose.

In both these cases, Craig and Jan complained of the 'identical' problem of painful, red, swollen knees. Yet when we look beyond the knees to what is taking place in the rest of the body, we see that these individuals have very different internal conditions. What they share in common is that both needed to have damp and heat cleared and eliminated from the channels that traverse the knee in order to cure the knee redness, swelling and pain. In Craig's case, however, internal heat also needed to be cleared, while in Jan's case, internal vacuity cold needed to be supplemented and warmed. If the treatment that was administered to Craig had been given to Jan, her condition would have worsened. Her weakened kidney and spleen yang would not have been able to handle the heat-clearing medicinals that Craig needed. The treatment Craig received would have weakened Jan's kidney and spleen yang causing her to feel even colder, exacerbating her loose stools (possibly causing diarrhoea) and creating even worse swelling in the legs which would have resulted in increased knee pain.

RHEUMATOID ARTHRITIS

The next two cases of rheumatoid arthritis also demonstrate how the same presenting problem, when looked at from the Chinese medical perspective, can have two different causes and approaches to treatment.

Cold in the channels with blood weakness

Rosa was a thin, athletic 29-year-old, single accountant who had received a positive diagnosis of rheumatoid arthritis (RA) the previous year. While Western medications were able to control her pain, she was worried about the long-term adverse effects on her health of using medications. A friend suggested she try Chinese medicine to see if it could help.

Rosa reported that her fingers would occasionally feel a little stiff. She had no bony changes in her hands or fingers. Since beginning the Western medications, the pain had been eliminated. Rosa's major complaint, beyond her diagnosis of RA and her stiff fingers, was her cold hands and feet. These were cold to the touch and had been so since her teenage years. Upon inquiry, it was found that she suffered from long menstrual cycles with sparse blood flow, dry skin, nails that easily split and hair that was dry and 'felt lifeless'.

According to Chinese medicine, Rosa's diagnosis was accumulation of cold in the channels with blood vacuity. Rosa had no yang vacuity symptoms like those of Jan above who had cold along with kidney and spleen yang vacuity. Rosa's symptom of long menstrual cycles with little blood indicated she had blood vacuity, especially in the light of her other blood vacuity symptoms. The blood is responsible for nourishing the skin, hair and nails. When the blood is vacuous or insufficient, the skin can be dry, nails can easily split and crack, and hair can lack lustre and life. In her case the blood was so vacuous and insufficient, it was unable to nourish her extremities (hands and feet). Cold had accumulated in the channels at the same time as her sinews became dried out due to malnourishment. The cold had caused her pain, but this had been eliminated by the Western medication. The remaining stiffness was a sign of stiff, dry sinews due to blood vacuity.

Rosa was given a famous Chinese herbal formula for nourishing and supplementing the blood. Called *Si Wu Tang* (Four Materials Decoction), its main ingredients are Radix Angelicae Sinensis (*Dang Gui*), cooked Radix Rehmanniae (*Shu Di*), Radix Albus Paeoniae Lactiflorae (*Bai Shao*) and Radix Ligustici Wallichii (*Chuan Xiong*). All these ingredients supplement and nourish the blood in Chinese medicine. To these, Caulis Milletiae Seu Spatholobi (*Ji Xue Teng*) was added to nourish the blood further while at the same time quickening the blood and eliminating any residual cold dampness. In addition, Radix Astragali Membranacei (*Huang Qi*) was added to boost the qi. It takes qi to engender and transform the blood. By adding a qi-supplementing ingredient, the blood-nourishing medicinals can work more quickly.

Rosa noticed a change in her stiff fingers within three days of beginning this formula. Her menses came earlier than she expected and the flow was heavier and longer. After taking this formula for two months, she reported that her nails no longer cracked and that her hair also seemed fuller and healthier. Chinese herbal medicine was a more effective treatment approach than acupuncture in Rosa's case as it is able to treat the blood directly.

Damp *bi*

Ken, 42, had been diagnosed with RA two weeks previous to our first meeting. An obese man, he was very anxious about his ability to continue his work as a graphic artist. The fingers on both hands were slightly swollen, stiff and sore. This made working as an artist difficult. Images of his aunt's crippled fingers haunted him. He experienced increased discomfort on cloudy, cold, rainy days. He had a numb and heavy sensation in both arms. When asked to describe his diet, he turned as red as a beetroot and said, 'I live on junk food.' Breakfast and lunch consisted of food purchased at a fast-food restaurant. Supper, which he ate with his wife, was a 'traditional meal': a main course of meat with some vegetable and bread followed by a sugary dessert. Ken's tongue was swollen and contained the imprints of his teeth on its borders, while its fur was thick, white and slimy looking. Ken's pulse was soggy and bowstring.

Ken's diagnosis was wind, cold, damp rheumatic *bi*. The primary pathogen was dampness. When damp settles into the channels, there will be stiffness, possible swelling, a heavy sensation and possible numbness. A further indicator of Ken's problem with damp was his weight, since, in Chinese medicine, fat is considered a problem of excessive dampness and phlegm. In addition, Ken's swollen tongue showed that he was not moving and transforming body fluids properly. The thick, white, slimy tongue fur showed that there was an accumulation of dampness, stagnant food, and possibly phlegm clogging his system. The soggy pulse showed that Ken's spleen was weak and that dampness was spilling over into the spaces between his muscles and flesh and his skin. This was obstructing the flow of qi and blood and so gave the pulse an image of constraint, a bowstring pulse.

Because Ken's dampness was due to poor spleen function resulting from a faulty diet, I instructed him on the principles of a clear, bland diet high in complex carbohydrates and fresh vegetables and low in sugars and sweets, dairy products, oils and fats, and uncooked and/or chilled foods and beverages. I also instructed him on the importance of regular exercise. I treated his sore, stiff, swollen fingers with acupuncture twice a week for several weeks. In addition, I prescribed a Chinese herbal formula which primarily supplemented the spleen and eliminated dampness.

Ken is still overweight and still does not eat what Chinese medicine would call a perfect diet. When work gets really stressful, Ken typically 'does not have time to eat right'. When that happens, his fingers swell up and become stiff and sore. When Ken eats correctly and gets regular exercise, he has no symptoms of his RA. During acute episodes, Ken comes back in to see me again. I do a couple of acupuncture treatments on his hands and give him another pep talk about diet and exercise. Otherwise, Ken is able to take care of himself and has continued to be able to practise his profession very successfully.

According to Western medicine, both Ken and Rosa had the same disease, rheumatoid arthritis. From the Chinese medical point of view, they had two completely different problems which required different treatments. Both patients were encouraged to incorporate a number of self-care suggestions into their daily routines. Rosa and Ken were encouraged to regulate their diets using the guidelines outlined in Chapter 10. They were advised to eat a more vegetarian diet and to eat primarily cooked foods. Both patients needed to improve their diets to strengthen their spleens. The spleen is responsible for the formation of blood (which was vacuous and insufficient in Rosa) and for moving and transforming dampness (which was excessive in Ken).

CONCLUSION

The cases presented above are but a sample of the complex spectrum of rheumatic diseases and the role Chinese medicine can play in their treatment. It is hoped that after reading these case histories and the multiple symptoms that accompany each person's pain you now have a feel for how a practitioner of Chinese medicine weaves together the many and various signs and symptoms to form a complete picture of the person — their Chinese medical pattern as opposed to their disease.

When speaking to a new patient, I often suggest that they write an 'obsessive' list of all their health complaints. Problems which seem unrelated to the disease may be relevant to the practitioner of Chinese medicine. With regard to recent injuries, the practitioner may focus primarily on the injury rather than going into other signs and symptoms in great depth. When dealing with stubborn, chronic conditions however, many details of the patient's health and bodily functions are important for making the diagnosis. Mental and emotional issues may also be highly relevant.

This is the beauty of Chinese medicine. It treats the whole person, not just the disease. Other aspects of health are likely to improve and there is healing with no side effects.

It is my hope that the case histories presented in this chapter will inspire you to consider having treatment with Chinese medicine. We will include details of how to find a qualified, local practitioner in a later chapter.

THE THREE FREE THERAPIES FOR ARTHRITIS AND RHEUMATIC COMPLAINTS

Most people reading this book will have grown up in a culture of Western medicine where an attitude prevails that it is the physician's job to diagnose and offer a cure. The patient has little responsibility other than to comply with treatment. Whilst this approach works well in some instances it is not always effective and sometimes we as patients need to make changes to our lifestyle in some way. Patients who suffer from heart conditions are often suddenly awakened to this reality; they need to make certain changes if they want to carry on living.

With chronic rheumatic conditions we may need to make changes to our lifestyle. This chapter will focus on these lifestyle changes from a Chinese medicine point of view. These changes really can make a difference; you can have less pain, be more mobile and rely less on medications.

CREATING THE CONDITIONS OF HEALING

I often use the phrase, 'creating the conditions of healing', to help people understand that they need to take an active role in their own health care. 'Creating the conditions of healing' is analogous to gardening. When we garden, we need to create a number of conditions so that our seeds will grow. First, we need to turn the soil over and fertilise it. Then we need to make sure that the garden gets the right amount of sun for the types of plants we are cultivating. We need to plant the seeds at the correct depth. We need to make certain that the seeds get enough water, but not too much. If these conditions are met, then we have done our job as gardener well. We've done everything possible to create the right conditions for the seeds to sprout and grow. At this point in the process, we wait for the miracle of life to unfold. All gardening, after the planting time, is waiting. We wait to see the plants come up through the soil. At that point, no amount of impatience, anger or demanding can change the outcome of our garden. And finally, when the seeds sprout, we may need to protect them from the wild world of weeds, birds, insects and all the other things that will do them harm.

Likewise we are the gardeners of our own life. We need to plant the seeds to create and promote a healthy, happy life. We need to nurture and protect ourselves from aspects of our lifestyle which could destroy our garden. If we create the right conditions and set the scene then nature's own healing powers will start to work more effectively. We have the potential in every moment to create the right conditions for healing.

It may be helpful to visualise our life and its many aspects as a flower, each petal representing an aspect of our life. To create the conditions of healing we need to make sure that each petal is nurtured and well cared for.

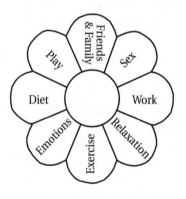

In this chapter we will explore the healing benefits of what I call the three free therapies. These are diet, exercise and deep relaxation and only you can take care of these three factors which are so important to your health and well-being.

DIET

In Chinese medicine, digestion is primarily a function of the spleen and stomach. Chinese dietary therapy is mostly concerned with promoting the healthy function of these two organs. The function of the spleen and stomach may be likened to cooking. The stomach receives the foods and liquids which then 'rot and ripen' like a mash in a fermentation vat. The spleen then cooks this mash and drives off (*i.e.*, transforms and sends upwards) the pure part. This pure part collects in the lungs to become the qi and in the heart to become the blood. All the principles of Chinese dietary therapy, including what persons with rheumatic complaints should and should not eat, are derived from these basic concepts.

As the spleen is the root of qi and blood production, keeping it functioning properly helps to ensure sufficient constructive and defensive qi. If the defensive qi is sufficient, it will protect the exterior of the body against invasion by the six environmental excesses. If the constructive and defensive qi are both sufficient, then the body will be properly warmed. Since warmth is one of the factors that promote and allow for the free flow of the qi and blood, having sufficient qi to warm the body is important for preventing the inhibited flow of qi and blood because of cold.

Secondly, healthy spleen function ensures that the blood production is sufficient. If the spleen does not create sufficient blood, the tissues of the body, including the sinews, will not receive adequate nourishment. The sinews may then dry up and become stiff. This would lead to stiffness and limitation in the range of movement of the joints surrounded by the sinews.

Thirdly, the spleen is in charge of moving and transforming body fluids. If the spleen becomes diseased and loses control over this function, fluids will collect and gather, transforming into dampness. Dampness may then spill over into the space between the muscles and skin, impeding the free flow of the qi and blood through the channels and vessels. Although dampness is one of the six environmental excesses, dampness which causes rheumatic *bi* conditions in the West is rarely just external dampness. If dampness endures in the body for a long time or is transformed by either cold or heat, it may congeal into phlegm. Phlegm is even denser than dampness, and obstructs the free flow of qi to an even greater extent than dampness.

Fourthly, because all the viscera and bowels of Chinese medicine form a single, interdependent whole, the function of the spleen is intimately connected to the function of all the other viscera and bowels. In particular, healthy spleen function ensures healthy liver and kidney function. If the spleen is strong and sufficient, then this helps the liver maintain its control over coursing and discharging, which, in turn, helps ensure the free flow of qi throughout the body. This ability of the spleen to control the liver has largely to do with the spleen's engendering sufficient blood to emolliate and harmonise the liver. As spleen qi and kidney yang are interdependent, spleen vacuity will eventually 'reach' the kidneys, leading to kidney yang vacuity. Since the kidneys govern the bones and joints, kidney vacuity can either cause or aggravate many types of joint pain. Although the spleen and kidneys both become debilitated by age (usually the spleen first, then, as a result, the kidneys), the spleen is the easier of the two viscera to supplement and strengthen via the diet. However, damage of the spleen due to an incorrect diet can speed up and exacerbate weakness and vacuity of the kidneys.

This is why a healthy, functioning spleen is of utmost importance in the prevention and treatment of all joint pain and rheumatic conditions. With regard to Chinese dietary therapy and the spleen, there are two main issues: 1) to avoid foods which damage the spleen, and 2) to eat foods which help build qi and blood.

Foods that damage the spleen

In terms of foods which damage the spleen, Chinese medicine begins with uncooked, chilled foods. If the process of digestion is likened to cooking, then cooking is really a pre-digestion outside the body. In Chinese medicine, it is thought that the majority of all foods should be cooked, *i.e.*, pre–digested. Although cooking may destroy some vital nutrients it does render the remaining nutrients much more easily assimilable. Thus, even though some nutrients have been lost, the net absorption of nutrients is greater with cooked foods than raw. It is thought that eating raw foods makes the spleen work harder and wears the spleen out more quickly. If one's spleen is very robust, eating uncooked, raw foods may not be so damaging, but we have already seen that many women's spleens are already weak because of their monthly periods overtaxing the spleen with regard to blood production. It is also a fact of life that the spleen typically becomes weak with age.

More importantly, chilled foods may directly damage the spleen. Chilled, frozen foods and drinks neutralise the spleen's yang qi. The process of digestion is the process of turning all foods and drinks to 100°F soup within the stomach so that it may undergo distillation. If the spleen expends too much yang qi simply to warm the food, then it will become damaged and weak. Therefore, all foods and liquids should be eaten and drunk at room temperature at least and better still at body temperature. The more signs and symptoms of spleen vacuity a person presents, such as fatigue, chronically loose stools, undigested food in the stools, cold hands and feet, dizziness on standing up and aversion to cold, the more they should avoid uncooked, chilled foods and drinks.

In addition sugary sweet foods may damage the spleen. Sweets are regarded as inherently damp-forming in Chinese medicine. Dampness is regarded as a yin pathogenic factor which if it becomes excessive will start to effect the yang qi in a negative way. The proper functioning of the spleen relies on yang qi. So sugary sweet foods if eaten to excess affect the spleen's ability to function properly.

Another group of foods which are dampening and, therefore, damaging to the spleen are what are known as 'sodden wheat foods'. This means flour products such as bread and noodles. Wheat (as opposed to rice) is damp by nature. When wheat is steamed, yeasted and/or refined, it becomes even more dampening. In addition, all oils and fats are damp by nature and, hence, may damage the spleen. The more oily or greasy a food is, the worse it is for the spleen. Because milk contains a lot of fat, dairy products are another spleen-damaging, dampness-producing food. This includes milk, butter and cheese.

If we put this all together, then ice cream is probably the worst thing a person with a weak, damp spleen could eat. Ice cream is chilled, it is intensely sweet, and it is filled with fat. Therefore, it is a triple whammy when it comes to damaging the spleen. Pasta smothered in tomato sauce and cheese is another recipe for disaster. Pasta made from wheat flour, tomatoes and cheese are all dampening. Additionally, what many people don't realise is that a glass of fruit juice contains as much sugar as many sweets, and is, therefore, very damp-producing and damaging to the spleen.

Below is a list of specific Western foods which are either uncooked, chilled, too sweet or too dampening and thus damaging to the spleen. Persons with rheumatic pain should minimise or avoid these according to how weak and damp their spleen is.

at the same time as it temporarily boosts the spleen, it does give a rush of yang qi. In addition, this rush of yang qi does move depression and stagnation, at least in the short term. So it makes sense that some people with liver depression, spleen vacuity and kidney yang debility might crave chocolate. That being said, the sugar in chocolate ultimately damages the spleen, and the oil causes or worsens dampness.

Alcohol
Alcohol is both damp and hot according to Chinese medical theory. It strongly moves the qi and blood. This means that with liver depression qi stagnation will feel temporarily better after drinking alcohol. However, the sugar in alcohol damages the spleen and creates dampness which blocks the flow of energy. The heat (yang) in alcohol can damage the blood (yin) and aggravate or inflame depressive liver heat. In particular, alcohol is contraindicated in any kind of damp heat condition.

Hot, peppery foods
Spicy, peppery, 'hot' foods also move the qi, thereby giving some temporary relief to liver depression qi stagnation. However, like alcohol, the heat in spicy hot foods adversely affects the blood and can inflame yang. Hot, peppery foods are specifically prohibited in damp heat patterns and conditions.

Sour foods
In Chinese medicine, the sour flavour is inherently astringent and constricting. People with liver depression qi stagnation should take care not to use too much vinegar and other intensely sour foods. Such sour-flavoured foods will only aggravate the qi stagnation by restricting the qi and blood all the more. An excess of sweet and sour foods such as orange juice and tomatoes is not advised for people with liver depression and spleen vacuity. This is because the sour flavour constricts the qi whilst the sweet flavour damages the spleen and creates

dampness. So, whenever there is a problem with the free flow of the qi and blood, it is best to limit or avoid an excess of sour foods, such as vinegar.

Diet drinks

I have found in practice that diet drinks or sodas seem to contain something that damages the Chinese concept of the kidney energy. They may not damage the spleen in the same way that sugary drinks do, but it doesn't mean that they are safe and healthy. I believe that diet drinks damage the kidney energies because a number of my patients over the years have reported that if they drink a lot of diet sodas, they experience urinary incontinence and soreness of the lower back and knees. When they stop drinking them these symptoms disappear. From the point of view of Chinese medical theory these are considered to be kidney vacuity symptoms. As women in their late 30s and throughout their 40s often have kidney vacuity signs I especially recommend that they steer clear of diet drinks. Anyone who has these signs of kidney vacuity or weakness which may often be present in cases of arthritis should ideally avoid diet drinks.

Foods which help nourish the blood

Qi and Wei

According to Chinese dietary therapy, all foods contain varying proportions of qi and *wei*. Qi means the ability to catalyse or promote yang function, while *wei* (literally meaning flavour) refers to a food's ability to nourish or construct yin substance. Since blood is relatively yin compared to qi being yang, a certain amount of food high in *wei* is necessary for a person to produce and transform blood. Foods which are high in *wei* as compared to qi are those which tend to be heavy, dense, greasy or oily, meaty or bloody. All animal products contain more *wei* than vegetable products. At the same time, black beans or, even better, black soya beans contain more *wei* than celery or lettuce.

When people suffer from joint pain due to blood vacuity failing to nourish the sinews, or yin vacuity failing to strengthen the bones, they usually need to eat slightly more foods high in *wei*. This includes animal proteins and products, such as meat and eggs. It is said that flesh foods are very 'compassionate' to the human body. This word recognises the fact that the animal's life has had to be sacrificed to produce this type of food. It also recognises that, because such food is so close to the human body itself, it is especially nutritious. This means that for people who suffer from vacuity rheumatic pain, eating some animal products is usually helpful and may sometimes be necessary.

Animal foods vs. vegetarianism

Based on my many years of clinical experience, I have seen many Westerners adhering to a strict vegetarian diet develop, after several years, blood or yin vacuity patterns. This is especially the case in women who lose blood every month and must build babies out of the blood and yin essence. When women who are strict vegetarians come to me with various complaints, if they present the signs and symptoms of blood vacuity, such as a swollen, pale tongue, pale face, pale nails, and pale lips, heart palpitations, insomnia, and fatigue with a fine, forceless pulse, I usually recommend that they include a little animal food into their diet. They often report back to me how much better they feel for this change in diet and how much more energy they have.

The downside of eating meat – besides the ethical issues – are that foods which are high in *wei* also tend to be harder to digest and to engender phlegm and dampness. Therefore, such foods should only be eaten in very small amounts at any one time. In addition, the weaker the person's spleen energy or the more phlegm and dampness they already have, the less *wei* foods they should eat in order to get the correct balance.

Remember that the process of digestion first consists of turning the food and drink ingested into 100°F soup in the stomach. Therefore, soups and broths made out of animal flesh are the easiest and most digestible way of adding some animal-quality *wei* to a person's diet. When eating flesh itself, this should probably be limited to only one to two ounces per serving and only three or four such servings per week. According to Chinese dietary theory, the best foods for creating and transforming blood and yin essence are organ meats and red or dark meats. This includes beef, venison, lamb, and dark meat from chicken, turkey, goose and duck. White meat fish and white meat fowl are less effective for building blood. White meat pork is also acceptable, as is ham.

One good recipe for adding more digestible *wei* to the diet of a person who is blood vacuous is to take a marrow bone and boil this with some cut vegetables, especially root vegetables, and black beans or black soya beans. Such a marrow bone, black bean and vegetable soup is easy to digest and yet rich in *wei*.

Food allergies, leaky gut, candidiasis and parasites

Western research suggests that many patients with systemic rheumatic diseases suffer from various food allergies. Often these food allergies are due to 'leaky gut syndrome'. This means the intestinal walls are more permeable than they should be. Hence they allow large, undigested food molecules into the bloodstream where they should not be and where they provoke allergic reactions. Frequently this type of leaky gut syndrome is due to or complicated by an overgrowth of yeast and fungi in the intestines. Everyone's intestines are home to many types of yeast and fungi. As long as their numbers stay in proportion to the protozoa and bacteria in the guts and as long as these fungi stay within the intestines themselves, there should be no problem. However, when they overgrow, they often move out of the intestines and into the body. They do so by sending out shoots or buds that wiggle through the intestines, thus causing leaks in the intestinal walls. Once inside the body, these fungi eventually die, and, when they decompose, their foreign proteins also provoke allergic reactions.

If the body is constantly fighting off foreign proteins, eventually two things happen. First, the body no longer recognises what it should and should not attack. Since the immune system loses its perspective due to being constantly overworked and revved up into high gear, it may start attacking the body's own healthy tissue. This is called an auto-immune response, and RA is classified as an auto-immune disease. Secondly, because the immune system is so overworked, it may not adequately protect the body against true foreign proteins and pathogens. Thus the body is continually invaded and assaulted, causing the immune system to become even more dysfunctional. In such cases, it is not uncommon to find that other amoebas and protozoa which are regarded as parasites are able to establish themselves within the guts. This only makes the intestinal flora and fauna more 'dysbiotic', meaning an unhealthy mix of intestinal populations, and hence the intestines function that much worse.

Food allergies, leaky gut syndrome, candidiasis and parasites are mostly Western medical concepts. Nonetheless, the signs and symptoms of all these are described in Chinese medicine. They are mainly associated with spleen vacuity and dampness, damp heat, liver depression and liver-kidney vacuities. Thus, an anti-candida diet is essentially the same as the Chinese 'clear, bland diet'.

Some last words on diet

In conclusion, Western patients are always asking me what they should eat in order to cure their disease. When it comes to diet, however, the issue is not so much what to eat as what not to eat. Diet most definitely plays a major role in the cause and perpetuation of many people's rheumatic complaints. Except in the case of vegetarians suffering from blood or yin vacuities, the key issue is what to avoid or minimise, not what to eat. Most of us know that coffee, chocolate, sugars and sweets, oils and fats, and alcohol are not good for us. Most of us know that we should be eating more complex carbohydrates and freshly cooked vegetables and less fatty meats. However, it's one thing to know these things and another to follow what we know.

To be perfectly honest, a clear, bland diet *à la* Chinese medicine is not the most exciting diet in the world. It is the traditional diet of our great-grandparents. Our modern Western diet, which is high in oils and fats, high in sugars and sweets, high in animal proteins, and proportionally high in uncooked, chilled foods and drinks, is a relatively recent development, and you can't fool Mother Nature.

When we change to the clear, bland diet of Chinese medicine we may at first suffer from cravings for more flavourful food. After a few days these cravings tend to disappear and we may be amazed that we don't miss some of our convenience or comfort foods as much as we thought we might. It is all too easy to become addicted to foods like sugar or caffeine that give us a short-term energy boost. Perseverance is the real key to long-term success. As the Chinese say, a million is made up of nothing but lots of ones, and a bucket is quickly filled by steady drips and drops.

EXERCISE

Exercise is the second of what are called the three free therapies. According to Chinese medicine, regular and adequate exercise has two basic benefits. First, exercise promotes the movement of the qi and quickening of the blood. Since all joint pain and rheumatic *bi* conditions by definition involve a lack of free flow, it is obvious that exercise is an important therapy for helping heal such *bi* conditions. Second, exercise benefits the spleen. The spleen's movement and transportation of the digestate is dependent upon the 'qi mechanism'. The qi mechanism describes the function of the qi in upbearing the pure and downbearing the turbid parts of digestion. For the qi mechanism to function properly, the qi must be flowing normally and freely. Since exercise moves and rectifies the qi, it also helps regulate and rectify the qi mechanism. This then results in the spleen's movement and transportation of foods and liquids and its subsequent engendering and transforming of the qi and blood. Because spleen vacuity typically complicates most chronic rheumatic complaints and because a healthy spleen checks and controls a depressed liver, exercise treats one of the other commonly encountered disease mechanisms in the majority of Westerners suffering from stubborn joint pain. Therefore, regular, adequate exercise is a vitally important component of any person's regime for either preventing or treating rheumatic complaints.

What kind of exercise is best?

In my experience, I find aerobic exercise to be the most beneficial for most people. By aerobic exercise, I mean *any* physical activity which raises your heartbeat 80% above its normal resting rate and keeps it there for at least 20 minutes. To calculate your normal resting heart rate, place your fingers over the pulsing artery on the front side of your neck. Count the beats for 15 seconds and then multiply by four. This gives you your beats per minute or BPM. Now multiply your BPM by 0.8. Take the resulting number and add it to your resting BPM. This gives you your aerobic threshold of BPM. Next engage in any physical activity you like. After you have been exercising for five minutes, take your pulse for 15 seconds once again at the artery on the front side of your throat. Again multiply the resulting count by four and this tells you your current BPM. If this number is less than your aerobic threshold BPM, then you know you need to exercise harder or faster. Once you get your heart rate up to your aerobic threshold, then you need to keep exercising at the same level of intensity for at least 20 minutes. In order to ensure that you are keeping your heartbeat high enough for long enough, you should recount your pulse every five minutes or so.

Depending on your age and physical condition, the amount of exercise you require to reach your aerobic threshold will vary. For some, simply walking briskly will raise your heartbeat 80% above its resting rate. Others will need to do more running, swimming, cycling or other more strenuous form of exercise. It doesn't really matter what the exercise is as long as it raises your heartbeat 80% above your resting rate and keeps it there for 20 minutes. However, there are two other criteria that you may wish to consider. First, the exercise should be something that is not too boring. If it is, then you may have a hard time keeping up your schedule. Second, the type of exercise should not cause any damage to any parts of the body. For instance, running on pavements may cause knee problems for some people. Therefore, you should pick a type of exercise you enjoy but also one which will not cause any problems or worsen your pain. For patients with joint or soft tissue pain, swimming or water aerobics can be an effective way to get a good cardiovascular workout without any damage.

When doing aerobic exercise, it is best to exercise either every day or every other day. If you do not do your aerobics at least once every 72 hours, then its cumulative effects will not be as great. I recommend that most of my patients do some sort of aerobic exercises every day or every other day, three to four times per week *at least.* The good news is that there is no real need to exercise more than 30 minutes at any one time. Forty-five minutes per session is not going to be all that much better than 25 minutes per session. And 25 minutes four times per week is very much better than one hour once a week.

Precautions during exercise

When a person has joint pain, it is important that the type of exercise undertaken does not further aggravate the injured or diseased joints. For instance, if one has *bi* pain in the knees, then running on a hard surface may actually make that pain worse. In that case, the pounding and stress of the running may only damage the tissues of the knees further, causing even more pain and inflammation which then retards the healing process. If this is the case, you will want to find an activity which either exercises those parts of the body which are not injured or which exercise the whole body without putting stress on the injured area. As mentioned previously, for those with injuries of the lower extremities, exercising in water can still mobilise the qi and blood without the injured part bearing the weight and stress of the body in normal gravity. The buoyancy of the water helps offset Earth's gravity, and you can mobilise the joints without causing further damage. Even if you cannot exercise the injured or diseased joint itself, you can usually still find some kind of exercise which will get your qi and blood flowing freely and smoothly.

DEEP RELAXATION

As we have seen above, rheumatic complaints are commonly associated with liver depression qi stagnation. Rheumatic *bi* and other types of joint pain keep us from doing what we want to do in our lives. In addition, the simple fact of pain is very stressful and irritating. Deep relaxation is therefore the third of our three free therapies. For deep relaxation to be therapeutic medically, it needs to be more than just mental equilibrium. It needs to be somatic or bodily relaxation as well as mental repose.

Even thoughts have an effect on our bodies and the way in which qi or energy moves. If we feel frustrated or stressed we may tense up, especially in the back, neck and shoulders. This then constricts the flow of qi and leads to liver depression and qi stagnation, which further constricts the flow of qi. In order to break this cycle we need to learn how to relax.

According to Chinese medicine each emotion is associated with a change in the direction of the flow of qi. Anger, for example, makes the qi move upwards, whilst fear makes the qi move downwards. Anger makes us feel as if we could blow our top or explode with anger. Fear may cause a sinking feeling; we feel paralysed or frozen with fear and in extreme circumstances we may urinate or defecate. All emotions are not just mental but bodily or somatic events. This is why it is important to clear your mind and relax your body at the same time.

Guided relaxation tapes

One of the most effective ways I have found for both myself and my patients to practise deep mental and physical relaxation is to use a guided progressive relaxation tape on a daily basis. Such tapes have a narrator who leads you through the process of relaxation allowing you to relax each part of the body progressively. There are many such tapes available these days through specialist shops. I recommend that you choose one or two that you feel comfortable with and enjoy listening to. In this way if you get bored of one you can go onto another.

Key things to look for in a good relaxation tape

There are four key things to look for to maximise the therapeutic effect of a good relaxation tape. Firstly, I would recommend that you ensure the tape is a guided tape and not a subliminal relaxation tape. Subliminal tapes usually have music and any instructions to relax are given so quietly that they are not consciously heard. Although such tapes can help you feel relaxed when you listen to them, ultimately they do not teach you how to relax as a skill which can be consciously practised and refined. Secondly, make sure the tape starts from the top of the body and works downwards. Remember, anger makes the qi go upwards in the body, and people with irritability and easy anger due to liver depression qi stagnation already have too much qi rising upward in their bodies. Such depressed qi typically needs to be moved downwards. Thirdly, make sure the tape instructs you to relax your physical body. If you do not relax all your muscles or sinews, the qi cannot flow freely and the liver cannot be coursed. Depression is not resolved, and there will not be the same medically therapeutic effect. And finally, choose a tape which instructs you to let your breath go with each exhalation. One of the symptoms of liver depression is a stuffy feeling in the chest which we then unconsciously try to relieve by sighing. Letting each exhalation go completely helps the lungs push the qi downward. This allows the lungs to control the liver at the same time as it bearsdown upwardly counterflowing angry liver qi.

GENTLE EXERCISE AND MEDITATION

More and more people these days are recognising the need to introduce some form of gentle exercise or meditation into their life. Gentle exercise can be beneficial in stretching the body and reducing stiffness. Meditation can help calm the mind which can be very helpful when dealing with physical pain. There are so many things now available for you to try, here are a few suggestions:

Yoga
Tai Chi
Qi Gong
Aikido and some
  martial arts

Meditation (whilst this can be a spiritual practice it can also provide an enormously beneficial and calming effect on the emotions)

The importance of daily practice
When I was an intern in Shanghai in the People's Republic of China, I was once taken on a field trip to a hospital clinic where they were using deep relaxation as a therapy for patients with high blood pressure, heart disease, stroke, migraines and insomnia. The doctors at this clinic showed us various graphs

plotting their research data on how such daily, progressive deep relaxation can regulate the blood pressure and body temperature and improve the appetite, digestion, elimination, sleep, energy and mood. One of the things they said has stuck with me for 15 years: 'Small results in 100 days, big results in 1,000.' This means that if one does such daily, progressive deep relaxation *every single day for 100 days*, one will definitely experience certain results. What are these 'small' results? These small results are improvements in all the parameters listed above: blood pressure, body temperature, appetite, digestion, elimination, sleep, energy and mood. If these are 'small' results, then what are the 'big' results experienced in 1,000 days of practice? The 'big' results are a change in how one reacts to stress — in other words, a change in one's very personality or character.

What these doctors in Shanghai stressed, and what I have also experienced both personally and with my patients, is that it is vitally important to do such daily, guided, progressive deep relaxation every single day, day in and day out for a solid three months at least and for a continuous three years at best. If one does such progressive, somatic deep relaxation every day, one will see every parameter or measurement of health and well-being improve. If one does this kind of deep relaxation only sporadically, missing a day here and there, it will feel good when you do it, but it will not have the marked, cumulative therapeutic effects that it could have. Perseverance is the real key to getting the benefits of deep relaxation.

The real test

Having a daily relaxation practice is really important but it's not the real goal. The ultimate goal is to learn how to deal with stress more effectively, breathing out and relaxing your body rather than holding your breath and tensing up. By doing such deep relaxation every day you will gradually learn how to recondition your body to stress. This is the real test, the game of life!

FINDING THE TIME

If you're like me and most of my patients, you are probably asking yourself right now, 'All this is well and good, but when am I supposed to find the time to eat well-balanced cooked meals, exercise at least every other day, and do a deep relaxation every day? I'm already stretched to the breaking point.' I know. That's the problem.

As a clinician, I often wish I could wave a magic wand over my patients' heads and make them all healthy and well. I cannot. After close to two decades of working with thousands of patients, I know of no easy way to health. There is good living and there is easy living. What most people take as the easy way these days is to continue pushing their limits continually to the maximum. The so-called path of least resistance will lead to problems in the long term. Unless you take time for yourself and find the time to eat well, exercise and relax, no treatment is going to eliminate your rheumatic complaints completely. There is simply no pill you can pop or food you can eat that will get rid of the root causes of most chronic disease: poor diet, too little exercise and too much stress. Even Chinese herbal medicine and acupuncture can only get their full effect if diet and lifestyle are first adjusted. Sun Si-maio, the most famous Chinese doctor of the Tang dynasty (618-907 CE), who himself refused government office and lived to be 101, said: 'First adjust the diet and lifestyle and only secondarily give herbs and acupuncture.' Likewise, it is said today in China, 'Three parts treatment, seven parts nursing.' This means that any cure is only 30% due to medical treatment and 70% is due to nursing, meaning proper diet and lifestyle.

In my experience, this is absolutely true. Seventy per cent of all disease will improve after three months of proper diet, exercise, relaxation and lifestyle modification. Seventy per cent! Each of us has certain non-discretionary rituals we perform each day. For instance, you may always and without exception find the time to brush your teeth. Perhaps it is always finding the time to shower. For others, it may be always finding the time each day to eat lunch. And for vast majority of us, we find the time to get dressed every day. The same applies to good eating, exercise and deep relaxation. Where there's a will there's a way. If your joint pain and rheumatic complaints are bad enough, you should find the time to eat well, get proper exercise and do a daily deep relaxation tape.

CONCLUSION

To see the real benefit of Chinese medicine it is vital to make the necessary changes to diet and lifestyle. Rheumatic complaints are not cured once and forever like measles or mumps. When I say Chinese medicine can cure joint pain, I do not mean that you will never experience unwanted pain in your joints again. What I mean is that Chinese medicine can eliminate or greatly reduce your symptoms *as long as you keep your diet and lifestyle together.* As a Chinese medicine practitioner, I try to give my patients an understanding of what causes their disease and what they can do to minimise or eliminate its causes and mechanisms. It is then up to them to decide what is an acceptable level of health.

CHINESE METHODS OF SELF-CARE FOR RHEUMATIC COMPLAINTS

I n the previous chapters we have seen how Chinese medicine treats joint pain, arthritis and rheumatic complaints with the help of a professional practitioner. We have also seen that diet, exercise and relaxation may all play an important role in helping with these conditions. One of the most important aspects of Chinese medicine is the emphasis it places on self-care. We will now look at a number of simple remedies that may be done at home.

Should you try any of these home remedies start slowly and cautiously and follow the directions given. If you experience any negative effects stop immediately and seek professional guidance.

QI GONG

Qi means the qi we have been talking about repeatedly throughout this book. *Gong* means to discipline or train. Therefore, *qi gong* exercises are exercises which train the qi. Although the words *qi gong* are no more than 100 years old, exercises for training the qi have been practised in China since at least 500 BCE. In the People's Republic of China today, there is a renaissance of interest in *qi gong*, with *qi gong* classes, books and research institutes sprouting up all over the place. Literally tens of millions of Chinese do some sort of *qi gong* every day. *Qi gong* can be done to promote health and prevent disease, while there are also *qi gong* exercises to treat almost every conceivable disease.

One simple *qi gong* exercise that anyone can do is to sit comfortably in a chair with your back straight. Breathing in, visualise the healing qi as a warm, milky light filling heaven above. Breathe this light in through the crown of your head as you inhale. Then as you exhale, visualise this light moving through your body to collect at the joint or joints which are affected. Imagine with each new breath that you are inhaling more and more healing qi from heaven. Then with each exhalation, wash the affected area in a bath of warm, healing qi and light. As you do this, feel the area become warm (as long as the condition is not a hot *bi*) and feel the qi moving to and through the affected area. Imagine that all the blockages are dissipated and that the area feels tingling with the effervescent feeling of flowing qi. One can continue like this for between several minutes and half an hour or more. At the end of the session, visualise that the affected area is completely healed, imagine that it is pain free, and that it is now ready to use again without limitation or disease.

If you suffer from hot *bi*, then feel this breath of life and light as a cool current bathing the affected area. Feel the congested heat dissipate and imagine that the swelling has dispersed.

To make this exercise even more powerful, you can pull the healing qi down from heaven with your hands on each inhalation, and then direct it to the affected joint or body part with the hands on the exhalation, thus mobilising the qi even more by coordinating the mind, breath, and the movement of the body.

There may be classes available locally in either *qi gong* or *t'ai chi*, which also cultivates and moves the qi. It can be very enjoyable and motivating to learn and practise with other people as well as at home.

CHINESE SELF-MASSAGE

Massage is a very effective way of stimulating the flow of energy and may therefore be very helpful for arthritic and rheumatic conditions.

We have included a self-massage regime here for peri-arthritis of the shoulder. This regime comes from a book by Fan Ya-Li entitled *Chinese Self Massage Therapy: The Easy Way to Health,* and it is available in the UK through Acumedic who are listed in the suppliers section.

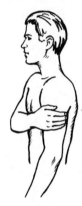

Begin by kneading the shoulder with the heel of the palm of the opposite hand. Knead every side of the affected shoulder, beginning with weak pressure and gradually applying stronger pressure. Do this for 3-5 minutes.

Next, pinch and grasp the muscles of the affected shoulder with the thumb, index and middle fingers of the other hand. Pinch and grasp all around the shoulder for 3-5 minutes, grasping more on the deltoid muscle on the side of the shoulder.

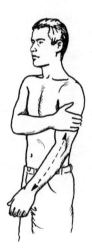

Now pinch and grasp the upper arm with the thumb, index and middle fingers of the other hand. Pinch and grasp the muscles on the front and back of the affected upper arm from the shoulder to the elbow 30-50 times.

This should be followed by pressing and kneading any particularly tender points around the affected shoulder, beginning with weak pressure and gradually pressing more and more strongly. At the same time, mobilise the shoulder. Do this for 2-3 minutes.

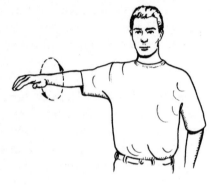

Rotate the affected shoulder joint in both directions approximately 10 times. Begin with small circles and increase to large circles.

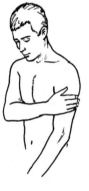

And finally, rub the shoulder and upper arm with the palm of the opposite hand, rubbing every side of the shoulder and upper arm until the whole area feels warm to the touch.

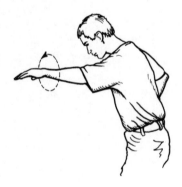

Now bend at the waist, stretch out the arm, and rotate the shoulder. The movement should start small and then gradually get larger. Likewise, the movement should start slowly and then gradually pick up speed.

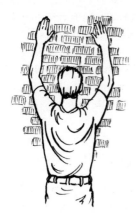

Stand facing a wall. With either both or only one hand, raise the arms as high as possible as if you were climbing the wall. Repeat this several times, increasing the height each time if possible.

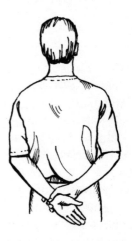

This regime is almost over when you bring both hands behind the body. With the healthy hand holding the wrist of the affected shoulder, lead the affected arm backwards as far as possible. Do this repeatedly several times.

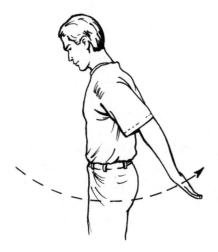

And finish up by swinging either both or only the affected arm backwards and forwards in an arc, making sure that the arm is very heavy and loose. By the time you finish, the shoulder should feel less stiff and painful and the whole arm should feel heavy, relaxed, tingling, warm and full of free-flowing qi.

Although a single self-massage treatment should make the affected joint or area feel better, self-massage is most effective when done on a regular basis every day for a number of days in a row. In this sense, the effects of Chinese self-massage are cumulative. Perseverance is therefore the key to getting good results with Chinese self-massage as it is with most of the self-help techniques suggested in this chapter.

MAGNET THERAPY

The Chinese have used magnet therapy since at least the Tang dynasty (618-907 CE). Placing magnets on the body is a powerful and painless way of stimulating acupuncture points. Since magnets can be taped onto points and 'worn' for days at a time, Chinese magnet therapy is able to provide easy, low-cost, continuous treatment. It is also possible to tape on magnets at night and to wear them to bed. There are many types of adhesive magnets available for stimulating acupuncture points.

Magnets range in strength from 400-9,000 gauss, the unit measuring magnetic strength. For the treatments below, I recommend you try 400-800 gauss magnets.

As magnet therapy can be very powerful I recommend that you seek professional advice should you experience any negative side effects from treatment.

The simplest way of using body magnets to free the flow of qi and blood in painful joints is to place a magnet with its south pole downwards on top of the skin directly over the most painful points. The more accurately you can locate these points, the better the result. In this case, there are two types of painful spots. The first is the most painful place when one moves the joint, while the second is found by pressing with the fingertips all around the soft tissue surrounding the point. Points which are painful when pressed are called *a shi* points in China, because a Chinese person will say '*a shi!*' ('That's it!') when the point is pressed.

Remember that all pain is a symptom of the lack of free flow of the qi and blood. Most rheumatic *bi* pain is due to either wind, cold, dampness, heat, phlegm or blood stasis obstructing the free flow of qi. According to Chinese medical theory, these blockages are all types of repletion. This means that they are something extra which should not be there. The principle for treating such 'repletions' in Chinese medicine is to drain them. The south side of a magnet is the draining side, while the north side is the supplementing side. If you first try the south side down on any *a shi* points and this makes the pain worse, try flipping the magnet over and put the north side down.

If the pain is vacuous or depleted in nature, meaning that it is worse after inactivity, at the end of the day, or when fatigued, the lack of free flow may not be due to anything blocking the channels and network vessels. Rather, it may be due to a simple lack of qi and blood to nourish and ensure the proper function of the sinews and vessels. In this instance, put the north side of the magnet down. In such 'vacuity' conditions, it is usually more difficult to find actual tender spots.

SEVEN STAR HAMMER

A seven star hammer is a small hammer or mallet with seven small needles embedded in its head. Nowadays in China, it is often called a skin or dermal needle and is also available in a single-use disposable version. It is one of the ways a person can stimulate various acupuncture points without actually inserting a needle into the body. Seven star hammers can be used either for people who are afraid of regular acupuncture, for children, or for those who wish to treat their condition at home. When the points to be stimulated are on the front of the body, this technique can be done by oneself. When they are located on the back of the body, this technique can be done by a family member or friend. This is a very easy technique which does not require any special training or expertise.

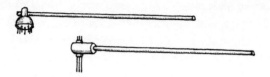

When treating joint pain with a seven star hammer, first wipe the affected area with rubbing alcohol or hydrogen peroxide to disinfect the skin. Then lightly tap all around the affected joint. If the condition is due to wind, cold and/or dampness, use medium strength and do not tap so hard as to cause any bleeding. The skin should simply become red in colour all around the affected joint or area. This redness is due to increased blood flow in this area. Since the qi is what moves the blood, seven star hammering like this stimulates the flow of both qi and blood.

If the condition is associated with blood stasis, damp heat or heat *bi*, then I do recommend tapping hard enough to cause not only redness of the skin but also a little light bleeding. Such bleeding helps drain static blood and/or pathogenic heat at the same time as it increases the flow of qi and blood locally. To avoid any possibility of infection, be sure to disinfect the area carefully after treatment, especially if you have caused any bleeding.

If there is lack of flow due to insufficiency of the qi and blood, then only tap very softly. This will help stimulate the qi and blood to move to and hence supplement and nourish the affected area. The basic rule of thumb with seven star hammering is that light tapping is supplementing, while heavy tapping is draining. The heavier the tapping the more draining this technique is.

Seven star hammering can be done on any individual joint in the body. It may also be done on top of and on either side of the spine. If there is neck joint pain, then one can tap all along the spine in the neck and the strap muscles to either side. Likewise, if there is low back pain, one can tap on top of the spine and on the long muscles to either side all up and down the affected area. This can be done either once or twice per day. Since this is not a very strong method of stimulation, like self-massage, it needs to be done consistently every day for a number of days in a row in order to see marked results.

After each treatment, the hammer should be soaked in rubbing alcohol or hydrogen peroxide in order to disinfect it between uses. Since these hammers are very inexpensive, I recommend that each person has their own and does not share them with others. Since you may cause a little bleeding doing this technique, you do not want to risk any cross-infection between persons sharing a single hammer. Slightly more expensive versions of these hammers are available made out of surgical steel. These can be boiled or cooked in a pressure cooker for 30 minutes to help sterilise them. Plastic versions can only be soaked in a disinfectant solution. Single-use disposable type 'hammers' are thrown away after each treatment.

THREAD MOXIBUSTION

Thread moxibustion refers to burning extremely tiny cones or 'threads' of aged Oriental mugwort (Folium Artemisiae Argyii, *Ai Ye*) directly on top of certain acupuncture points. When done correctly, this is a very simple and effective way of strongly stimulating the flow of qi and blood and adding yang qi to the body without causing a burn or scar.

To do thread moxa you will need to buy the finest grade of Japanese moxa wool — it is called Japanese pure moxa — and very thin incense or akabane sticks to light it with. Pinch off a tiny amount of the moxa and roll it between your first finger and thumb to produce a thick 'thread'. Pinch a small amount of the thread off so you have something the size of a sesame seed. This should then be placed on the chosen point — you will probably need to wet the point with water or apply petroleum jelly to make the moxa stick to it. See illustration on page 103 for further detail. The moxa thread should be upright with a narrow part at the top and bottom where it touches the skin. Light the thread with the incense stick. As soon as you start to feel anything then extinguish the moxa thread by pressing down on it firmly with a finger. The thread is so small that it will be quickly put out and your finger should not get burnt. The trick is to be confident and firm about putting it out. If you do get burnt try applying lavender essential oil to the burn to promote rapid healing. Repeat the whole procedure starting with three or four threads on the point per daily treatment and building up to ten. The rapid heat on the painful point is a very effective way of moving the energy and qi blockage.

For many sufferers of arthritic or rheumatic conditions, treating the affected area alone will not be enough. You will need to boost the underlying vacuity or deficiency within the body's energy before the pain and symptoms may be relieved. There are three points on the body that are very powerful for stimulating an overall deficiency or vacuity, especially when moxa is applied to them. They are called Sea of Qi, First Gate and Leg Three Miles according to English translation. Even the names of these points conjure up images of energy and vitality. For this treatment I recommend large moxa cones which are made of either Japanese semi-pure moxa or the finest grade of Chinese moxa. The moxa wool should be formed into large cones with a base size of one or two centimetres. The cone is then briefly floated in a glass of water to wet the base and then placed on the chosen point and lit; you should remove it as soon as you feel any warmth and quickly place it in a glass of water to extinguish it. Repeat for three to five cones on each point. In Japan this technique is called *Chinetsukyu* moxa. It is very beneficial for boosting the energy: the gentle warming is more effective for supplementing a deficiency than the rapid heat of thread moxa on local points which is a more 'moving' treatment. I recommend that you do this treatment daily for a week or two and see if it is beneficial for you in terms of general health and well-being.

Moxibustion is not an appropriate treatment for everyone and may not be advisable in some instances of high blood pressure. If you decide to try moxibustion and you experience any negative effects then stop the treatment and seek professional advice.

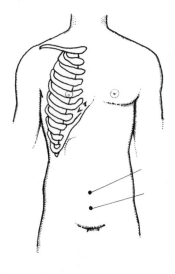

Qi Hai (Conception Vessel 6) English name – Sea of Qi: This point is located two finger-breadths below the navel on the midline of the lower abdomen. It supplements the qi of the entire body.

Guan Yuan (Conception Vessel 4) English name – First Gate: This point is located four finger-breadths below the navel on the midline of the lower abdomen. It especially supplements the yang qi and essence of the kidneys.

Zu San Li (Stomach 36) English name –
Leg Three Miles: This point is located
three finger-breadths below the lower,
outer corner of the kneecap in a
depression between the muscles on
the lateral side of the lower leg. It
supplements the creation and
transformation of the qi and blood of
the entire body via the spleen and
stomach.

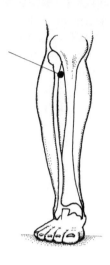

Although these points are quite easy
to locate, I recommend visiting a local
professional acupuncturist so that they
can teach you how to do this technique
safely and effectively and how to locate
these three points accurately.

MOXA STICK

A moxa stick is another way of using aged Oriental mugwort
(Folium Artemisiae Argyii, *Ai Ye*) to increase the flow of qi and
blood in the treatment of arthritis or rheumatic complaints. In
this case the moxa *does not touch the skin* but is held over or
under specific acupuncture points or areas of pain. This method
is especially effective in cases of yang vacuity cold pain where
the discomfort is clearly improved by warmth. There may also
be other symptoms of vacuity cold such as cold feet or legs,
abdominal pain which is improved by warmth, excessive
urination, a pale or bluish tongue, or a slow, deep pulse.

To use this method of moxibustion, you should light the
moxa stick and hold it over or under the affected areas of pain
for several minutes until the skin has turned quite pink, usually
five to seven minutes. Be careful not to burn the skin. When the
heat feels scorching, move the stick away for a few seconds and
then back again. You can use a chicken-pecking motion,

repeatedly moving the stick closer to the skin and then farther away, or a circular motion, going around and around the area to be treated. This can be done at any joint, although it should not be administered over the heart, on the face, over the external genitalia, or on the centre of the back just behind the heart.

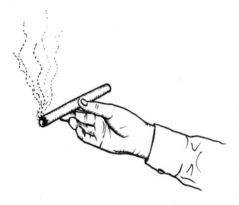

Moxa sticks are now available in a smokeless version which can be useful if you are sensitive to smoke. The smoke itself is considered to have therapeutic value in Chinese medicine.

A moxa stick treatment can be used every day or every other day. If you are unsure about these instructions, a local acupuncture practitioner can instruct you in the correct use of this type of therapy. As with any of these suggestions, if the use of moxa seems to be making your symptoms worse, discontinue immediately and seek professional advice.

HYDROTHERAPY

Hydrotherapy means water therapy and is also a part of traditional Chinese medicine. There are several different water treatments for helping relieve joint pain and rheumatic complaints. If dampness is the major obstructing factor in your rheumatic compliant, then you probably will not choose hydrotherapy as a major part of your healing regime. However, if wind, cold or heat are the major factors, then you can use hydrotherapy safely and effectively. It is also possible to use hydrotherapy if dampness is only a contributory or secondary factor.

As we have seen above, heat is yang and yang is associated with movement and transformation. When the body obtains warmth, the qi and blood flow more freely and easily. Although Western medicine, looking inside the body microscopically, says that the tissues are inflamed in most rheumatic complaints, that does not mean that applying ice is really a good idea. The Chinese practitioner does not look inside the joint, but rather infers what is going on inside from what manifests on the outside. Unless there is redness and heat on the outside of the body, the practitioner is probably going to recommend warm applications rather than cold. Cold is yin and, therefore, is associated with stillness and contraction. When the body obtains cold, that cold inhibits and congeals the flow of qi and blood. Since pain implies lack of free flow already, except in cases of very recent traumatic injury with marked redness and heat or in cases of hot *bi*, Chinese practitioners always choose warm-water applications for the treatment of rheumatic complaints.

For acute joint pain due to wind, cold or damp *bi*, you should heat some water and soak a cotton towel in it. Wring it out and apply to the affected area. The towel should be as hot as possible without burning the body. Cover with another dry towel and keep in place for 15 minutes. Do this once every hour. After removing this hot compress, rub some very cold water over the surface briefly in order to close the pores. This will keep any further external excesses from invading and settling in the affected area. Then cover the body and be sure not to get chilled.

For acute joint pain due to heat *bi* or damp heat *bi*, dip a cotton cloth in cold water and wrap loosely around the affected area. Pin this in place but be sure that the cloth is loose. Do not make the cloth so tight that it constricts the joint and cuts off the flow of qi and blood. We want the qi and blood to flow through the area as freely as possible. However, we also need to clear the heat. In order to clear heat and reduce inflammation, sprinkle some cold water on the cloth every 15 minutes or so to keep the compress continuously cold.

For chronic joint pain, warm-water soaks, hot baths or steam baths are recommended. Generally, you should continue the hot-water treatment for at least 20 minutes at a time. However, you should not stay in the hot water or steam bath for more than a maximum of two hours at any given time. As with acute joint pain, warm-water applications for chronic rheumatic complaints should be followed by a very brief application of cold water in order to close the pores. Similarly, you must bundle up and stay warm afterwards so as to avoid further invasion.

For chronic joint pain it is also possible to spray the affected area with hot water for several minutes. The more pressure, the better. Many modern shower heads allow for a focused stream of water under some pressure. Then switch to 15 seconds of intensely cold water. Alternate back and forth like this several times, always using the hot water for a long time and the cold water for a very short duration, always beginning with warm water and finishing with a very short application of cold.

CHINESE HERBAL REMEDIES FOR HOME THERAPY

In this next section I will give some recipes which you can make at home in the form of wines, porridges and teas. As with all Chinese herbs I strongly recommend that you seek professional guidance with regard to their usage. You will probably need to go through a qualified practitioner to obtain the herbs in the UK, as reputable suppliers do not sell to the general public. You may also find that not all the ingredients are available in the UK, in which case your practitioner may be able to recommend alternatives. Some of the ingredients are simple food stuffs and may not require a prescription. Should you choose to try one of these recipes and notice any unwanted side-effects, stop taking it immediately and seek advice from your practitioner.

Chinese herbal wines

In Chinese medicine alcohol is said to quicken the healing effects of other herbs. It is also very effective for moving the blood and qi. A number of Chinese medicinal wines can help with bi conditions such as arthritis, joint pain and rheumatism although some people with an auto-immune disorder may be advised not to drink alcohol. Medicinal wines can easily be made at home and some may be available in specialist Chinese shops in Chinatown. Alcohol is considered to be hot in Chinese medicine so it is best used if the bi condition involves cold. It is also good in the winter when the weather is cold. In China, medicinal wines are especially popular with the elderly.

Dang Gui Song Ye Jiu (Angelica Sinensis and Pine Needles Wine) This wine scatters wind, dispels cold and quickens the blood. It is indicated for wind cold *bi* complicated by blood stasis. It is made by taking two big handfuls of fresh pine needles and Radix Angelicae Sinensis (*Dang Gui*), 150g/6oz. Put these ingredients in a litre of brandy or vodka and allow to steep for six to seven weeks. At the end of that time, remove the dregs and reserve the liquid. Drink this medicinal wine when you feel the pain.

Hei Dou Qiang Huo Jiu (Black Soya Bean and Notopterygium Wine) This wine resolves the exterior and tracks down wind, overcomes dampness and stops pain. It is indicated for wind damp *bi* possibly complicated by blood vacuity not nourishing the sinews. Thus there is joint pain and especially stiffness accompanied by a pale face, pale lips, pale nails, pale tongue, dry skin and dry hair. The ingredients in this wine are Radix Et Rhizoma Notopterygii (*Qiang Huo*), 15g/1tbsp, Radix

Ledebouriellae Divaricatae (*Fang Feng*), 10g/2tsp, and dry fried black soya beans (*Hei Dou*), 30g/2tbsp. Grind the above three ingredients into powder in a coffee grinder and soak in 200ml/7oz of rice wine or sake. Allow to soak for one week and then drink a small amount each evening either before or after dinner.

Dan Shen Du Zhong Jiu (Salvia and Eucommia Wine)
This wine quickens the blood and opens the network vessels, nourishes the liver and supplements the kidneys. It is used to treat blood stasis with simultaneous liver blood and kidney yin and/or yang vacuity. Mostly this manifests as chronic low back and lower extremity pain in older patients. Its ingredients are Cortex Eucommiae Ulmoidis (*Du Zhong*), 60g/2¼oz, Radix Salviae Miltiorrhizae (*Dan Shen*), 60g/2¼oz, and Radix Ligustici Wallichii (*Chuan Xiong*), 40g/1½oz. Grind these into powder and place in a large jar. Cover with a litre of vodka or brandy and allow to soak for five to seven days. Then remove the dregs and drink a small amount every evening either before or after dinner.

Ling Pi Di Huang Jiu (Epimedium and Rehmannia Wine)
This wine supplements the kidneys and invigorates yang, dispels wind and dampness, and strengthens the sinews and bones. It treats lack of strength and pain of the low back and chronic wind damp *bi* in patients with a vacuous constitution or in the elderly. Its ingredients are Herba Epimedii (*Xian Ling Pi*), 250g/9oz, and cooked Radix Rehmanniae (*Shu Di*), 150g/5oz. Grind the above two ingredients and soak them for five to seven days in two litres of vodka or brandy. Drink some of this each evening either before or after dinner.

If you prefer your alcohol a little sweeter, then use brandy as the tincturing agent. If you prefer your alcohol drier, then use vodka. If you do not like or cannot tolerate strong spirits, then use sake or rice wine.

Chinese herbal teas

Here are some recipes for teas which may be helpful for *bi* conditions. These or similar alternatives are available from some herbal suppliers although a prescription from a qualified herbal medicine practitioner is required in the UK.

Jiang Can Liang Jiang Cha (Bombyx and Alpinia Tea)
This tea scatters cold, dispels wind and stops pain. It can be used to treat wind, cold, damp *bi* pain. Its ingredients are equal amounts of Bombyx Batriticatus (*Jiang Can*), Rhizoma Alpiniae Officinari (*Gao Liang Jiang*) and green tea. Grind these three ingredients into fine powder and store in a dry place. To use, take 3g/½tsp of this powder and steep in a cup of boiling water. This tea can be drunk two or three times per day.

Du Huo Cha (Angelica Pubescens Tea)
This tea is made from a single ingredient, Radix Angelicae Pubescentis (*Du Huo*). Boil 20g/¾oz of this herb in water, remove the dregs and drink freely throughout the day as tea. It dispels wind, scatters cold and disinhibits dampness. It is used to treat wind, damp, cold *bi* pain in the joints, especially if this pain wanders about from joint to joint.

Mu Gua Cha (Chinese Quince Tea)
This tea soothes the sinews and quickens the network vessels, harmonises the stomach and transforms dampness. It can be used for bone and joint pain primarily due to damp *bi* and primarily in the lower part of the body. It is made by taking Fructus Chaenomelis Lagenariae (*Mu Gua*), 15–20g/3–4tsp, Cortex Radicis Acanthopanacis (*Wu Jia Pi*), 12g/2tsp, and honey mix-fried Radix Glycyrrhizae (*Zhi Gan Cao*), 6g/1tsp, and boiling these in 500ml/17 fl oz of water for 15 minutes. Drink this tea. You can reboil the herbs in order to make more liquid if necessary.

Yi Mi Fang Feng Cha (Coix and Ledebouriella Tea)
This tea dispels wind and eliminates dampness. It treats heaviness, swelling, and soreness due to damp *bi*. It consists of Semen Coicis Lachryma-jobi (*Yi Yi Ren*), 30g/2tbsp, and Radix Ledebouriellae Divaricatae (*Fang Feng*), 10g/2tsp. Boil these two medicinals in water and drink as a tea, one packet per day. This tea is also suitable if there is a slight amount of heat as well as dampness as evidenced by slight redness and slight heat in the affected joint.

Gu Sui Bu Cha (Drynaria Tea)
This tea is made out of Rhizoma Drynariae (*Gu Sui Bu*), 50g/2oz, and Ramulus Cinnamomi Cassiae (*Gui Zhi*), 15g/1tbsp. These are boiled in water and the resulting beverage drunk warm throughout the day. Use one packet each day. This tea quickens the blood and scatters cold, supplements the kidneys and strengthens the low back. It can be used to treat low back sprain as well as chronic low back pain due to kidney vacuity and/or blood stasis.

Chinese herbal porridges

As with Chinese medicinal wine and teas, there is a whole repertoire of medicinal porridges within Chinese medicine. Sometimes called congee, these medicinal porridges are made with a grain, usually rice, and one or two Chinese herbs. Because everything that is eaten must be transformed into 100°F soup before any further digestion and assimilation can begin, soups and porridges are an especially healthy way of eating. When such soups and porridges are made with Chinese herbs as part of their ingredients, then truly medicinals and food have a common source. Below are several Chinese medicinal porridge recipes which can be used for the treatment of rheumatic complaints.

Wu Dou Zhou (Black Bean Congee)

This porridge is made from black soya beans, 30g/2tbsp, white or brown rice, 100g/4oz, and a little brown sugar to taste unless one suffers from hypoglycaemia or candidiasis and is thus very sensitive to any sugar at all. Soak the black soya beans in water overnight. Then cook the beans and rice into a porridge in one litre of water. Eat once or twice each day. This congee helps expel wind and quicken the blood, disinhibits dampness and disperses swelling. It can be used for wind damp *bi* with swelling, heaviness and soreness of the joints.

Yi Mi Zhou (Coix Congee)

This porridge only consists of a single ingredient, Semen Coicis Lachryma-jobi (*Yi Yi Ren*). Take 50g/2oz of Coix or Job's tears barley and cook with a suitable amount of water to make a thin gruel. As long as one is not overly sensitive to sugar, one may add just a little brown sugar to taste. This congee fortifies the spleen and eliminates dampness and can also be used to treat damp *bi*. Although Coix does not clear heat, it can be used to treat damp heat *bi* as a support to other treatment which will help clear the heat.

Cang Er Zi Zhou (Xanthium Seed Congee)

This porridge dispels wind and scatters cold, brightens the eyes, sharpens the hearing and opens a blocked nose. It can be used to treat wind, cold, damp *bi* as well as headache, stuffy nose and toothache. It is made from Fructus Xanthii Sibirici (*Cang Er Zi*), 15g/1tbsp and white or brown rice, 50g/2oz. First dry-fry the Xanthium seeds till they turn yellow. Then boil them in 200ml/7oz of water down to 100ml/3½fl oz of liquid. Add this liquid to the rice along with another 400ml/14 fl oz of water and cook the rice into porridge. Eat this warm twice a day.

Da Ma Zhou (Cannabis Congee)
This porridge is made out of Semen Cannabis Sativae (*Huo Ma Ren*), 10g/2tsp, and white or brown rice, 50g/2oz. The cannabis seeds have been heat treated to prevent germination. First mash the Cannabis seeds and boil them in water. Afterwards, add the resulting liquid to the rice and cook it into a thin gruel. Eat once each morning and night. This congee moistens the intestines and quickens the blood. It can help treat wind *bi* complicated by blood vacuity dryness. This manifests as constipation, pallor and inhibition of the joints which are especially stiff.

Ye Jiao Teng Zhou (Polygonum Vine Congee)
This porridge nourishes the blood and quiets the spirit, dispels wind and frees the flow of the network vessels. It can be used to treat restlessness, insomnia and dream-disturbed sleep but also wind damp *bi* conditions. It is made by cooking 50g/2oz of white or brown rice with two Red Dates (Fructus Zizyphi Jujubae, *Da Zao*), and 60g/2¼oz of Caulis Polygoni Multiflori (*Ye Jiao Teng*). First decoct the Polygonum in 500ml/14 fl oz of water, remove the dregs, and add the resulting liquid to the rice and Red Dates. Add another 200ml/7 fl oz of water and cook into porridge. Eat warm one hour before bed each evening for insomnia. As long as you do not react badly to sugar, you can add a little brown sugar or honey to taste.

Chinese herbal liniments and plasters
There are a number of different ready-made Chinese plasters for use in the treatment of rheumatic complaints and joint pain.

These or similar alternatives are available from some herbal suppliers although a prescription from a qualified herbal medicine practitioner is required in the UK. The suppliers may be able to suggest alternatives which don't require a prescription.

Jing Zhi Gou Pi Gao (Manufactured Essence Dog Skin Plaster, simply called Rheumatic Plaster on the box)

This is one of the very common adhesive plasters manufactured in China for the local topical treatment of rheumatic complaints. Traditionally, a herbal paste was smeared on dog skin in order to make healing poultices. However, nowadays, you may be relieved to hear, adhesive-backed cotton plasters impregnated with Chinese herbal extracts are used instead. Only the name 'dog skin' remains. The ingredients in this popular plaster are intended to penetrate through the skin aromatically and move the qi strongly and quicken the blood. These plasters can be used for any kind of rheumatic or traumatic pain. They are not specific to wind, damp, cold or heat *bi*.

Apply one plaster over the area of pain and leave in place for 24 hours. A single plaster can also be cut into two or more smaller plasters to cover smaller areas. Do not wear in the bath or shower. Do not apply over open wounds or skin lesions. If the plaster causes a blister or other skin irritation, remove it at once. As long as the area stays irritated, it will actually continue to promote healing of the underlying tissues. This is called 'counter-irritation' and is a very old medical principle used all over the world.

She Xiang Zhui Feng Gao (Musk Expelling Wind Plaster)

This plaster also contains strongly aromatic and penetrating medicinals that move the qi and quicken the blood. Like the plaster above, it is non-specific for various types of impediment as well as for blood stasis pain. Apply and use in the same way as above.

Shang Shi Zhi Tong Gao (Damage Due to Dampness, Stop Pain Plaster)

This plaster works in the same way as the preceding two. Although it contains the word dampness in its name, in fact it can be used for any type of *bi* or blood stasis due to traumatic injury. Apply and use as above. Another product with a similar name is *Shang Shi Bao Zhen Gao* (Damage Due to Dampness Protect the True Plaster).

Shen Xian Jin Bu Huan Gao (Magic Immortal Not To Be Exchanged for Gold Plaster, also simply called Magic Plaster)
This plaster can be used for wind, cold, damp *bi* or for blood stasis. It consists of a large glob of hardened herbs on a cloth backing. The herbs are mixed with beeswax. To use, you can either steam the plaster until the wax softens or put it in an oven on low to warm it up and melt the wax. When the wax has become soft, apply the plaster to the affected area. However, take care not to apply it too hot or it will cause a nasty burn. If the plaster falls off, heat it up a second time and use it again. If the skin becomes irritated or the plaster causes blistering, remove and discontinue its use.

Bao Xin An You (Protect the Peace of the Heart Oil, also called *Po Sum On* Medicated Oil)

This medicated oil can be applied topically to the affected joint or body part. It contains similar aromatic, penetrating, qi-moving and blood-quickening ingredients to the above plasters. It can be used for wind, cold, damp *bi* or blood stasis joint pain and rheumatic complaints. It is often used with either Chinese self-massage or professionally administered Chinese medical massage. Apply directly to the skin liberally and often. Do not get in the eyes. Wash the hands after application, and do not touch the genitalia while this oil is still on the hands. This oil will stain one's clothes, but it can be removed with rubbing alcohol.

All the plasters and liniments discussed above are ready-made and can be purchased from appropriate sources. Below are several recipes for liniments which you can make in your own home.

Shao Lin Wu Xiang Jiu (Shaolin Five Fragrances Wine)

The Shaolin Monastery is famous in Chinese lore for being the home of esoteric martial and healing arts. The following recipe is an authentic one from the Shaolin Monastery. It quickens the blood and scatters stasis, disperses swelling and stops pain. It can be used to treat traumatic injuries as well as wind, damp, cold *bi* conditions. Its ingredients consist of: Flos Caryophylli (*Ding Xiang*), 9g/2tsp, Radix Auklandiae Lappae (*Mu Xiang*), 9g/2tsp, Resina Olibani (*Ru Xiang*), 9g/2tsp, Lignum Santali Albi (*Bai Tan Xiang*), 9g/2tsp, Fructus Foeniculi Vulgaris (*Xiao Hui Xiang*), 9g/2tsp, Radix Angelicae Sinensis (*Dang Gui*), 30g/2tbsp, Radix Ligustici Wallichii (*Chuan Xiong*), 24g/1oz, Lignum Sappan (*Su Mu*), 24g/1oz, Radix Achyranthis Bidentatae (*Niu Xi*), 24g/1oz, Flos Carthami Tinctorii (*Hong Hua*), 15g/1tbsp. Place these ingredients in a large-lidded pot or jar. Add 500ml/14 fl oz of rubbing alcohol and allow to steep for one month, shaking often. After one month, remove the dregs and bottle for use. Apply topically to the affected area several times a day.

Other liniment recipes
These liniment recipes are strictly for external application.

1. Take Resina Myrrhae (*Mo Yao*), 3g/1tsp, Resina Olibani (*Ru Xiang*), 3g/1tsp, Lacca Sinica Exsiccata (*Shan Qi*), 3g/1tsp, Flos Carthami Tinctorii (*Hong Hua*), 3g/1tsp, Borneol (*Bing Pian*), 0.8g/¼tsp, Radix Auklandiae Lappae (*Mu Xiang*), 1g/¼tsp, Camphor (*Zhang Nao*),* 6g/1tsp, Sanguis Draconis (*Xue Jie*),

---

* Camphor may be more readily available from a Western rather than Chinese herbal supplier.

9g/2tsp, and soak in one litre of rubbing alcohol for two weeks. Remove the dregs and bottle for use. Apply topically to the affected area for the treatment of blood stasis due to traumatic injury as well as for pain due to wind, cold, damp *bi.*

2. Take 30g/2tbsp each of Flos Carthami Tinctorii (*Hong Hua*), Radix Aconiti (*Chuan Wu*), Radix Aconiti (*Cao Wu*)**, Extremitas Radicis Angelicae Sinensis (*Dang Gui Wei*), Semen Pruni Persicae (*Tao Ren*), Radix Glycyrrhizae (*Gan Cao*), uncooked Rhizoma Zingiberis (*Sheng Jiang*), Herba Ephedrae (*Ma Huang*)***, Semen Strychnotis (*Ma Qian Zi*), Ramulus Cinnamomi Cassiae (*Gui Zhi*), Radix Auklandiae Lappae (*Mu Xiang*) and Resina Myrrhae (*Mo Yao*) and put in a large-lidded jar or bottle. Add 1l/1¾pt of rubbing alcohol and allow to soak for two weeks. Shake often. Then remove the dregs and bottle for use. Apply topically to the affected area. *Do not use internally!* This liniment is better for wind, cold, damp *bi* and not as good for traumatic injuries as the previous formula.

3. Take Herba Ephedrae (*Ma Huang*)***, 21g/¾oz, Ramulus Mori Albi (*Sang Zhi*), 9g/2tsp, Radix Ledebouriellae Divaricatae (*Fang Feng*), 6g/1tsp, Zaocys Dhumnades (*Wu Shao She*), 12g/2½tsp, Bombyx Batryticatus (*Tian Chong*), 3g/½tsp, Flos Carthami Tinctorii (*Hong Hua*), 15g/1tbsp, Radix Aconiti (*Chuan Wu*)**, 9g/2tsp, Radix Angelicae Dahuricae (*Bai Zhi*), 6g/1tsp, Radix Et Rhizoma Notopterygii (*Qiang Huo*), 3g/½tsp, Radix Angelicae Pubescentis (*Du Huo*), 3g/½tsp, Cortex Radicis Dictamni Dasycarpi (*Bai Xian Pi*), 6g/1tsp, Herba Siegesbeckiae (*Xi Xian Cao*), 9g/2tsp and soak in one litre of rubbing alcohol for two weeks. This liniment is suitable for wind, damp, cold *bi* which is more deep-seated and chronic than the above.

** Radix Aconiti is a restricted substance in the UK and you may have difficulties obtaining it.

*** Herba Ephedrae is not available except for professional use in the UK.

Chinese herbal soaks

And finally, it is also possible to treat various painful joints and body parts due to wind, damp, cold *bi* by immersing the affected joint or body part in a hot medicinal soak. One such soak can be made by taking 9g/2tsp each of Radix Et Rhizoma Notopterygii (*Qiang Huo*), Radix Angelicae Pubescentis (*Du Huo*), Resina Olibani (*Ru Xiang*), Resina Myrrhae (*Mo Yao*), Radix Aconiti (*Chuan Wu*)*, Radix Aconiti (*Cao Wu*), Herba Lycopodii Cernui (*Shen Jin Cao*), Ramulus Cinnamomi Cassiae (*Gui Zhi*), Fructus Cheanomelis Lagenariae (*Mu Gua*), Fructus Liquidambaris Taiwaniae (*Lu Lu Tong*), Rhizoma Acori Graminei (*Shi Chang Pu*), Eupolyphaga Seu Ophistoplatia (*Tu Bie Chong*) and Flos Carthami Tinctorii (*Hong Hua*). Boil these ingredients in a big pot of water for 15-30 minutes. Remove the dregs and allow to cool to the hottest temperature you can bear without burning yourself. Soak the affected area for 15 minutes. Then be sure to dry and cover the affected area afterwards so that it does not become chilled. This can be done once or twice a day. The same medicinals can be reboiled for several days in a row before changing to fresh ones. This method is especially good for treating either hand or foot *bi*.

LEARNING TO LIVE WITH PAIN

Sadly not all pain is curable. The painful sensations in our body ebb and flow. When our attention is continually focused on pain and how we may rid ourselves of it, our world becomes very small. Our pain becomes the centre of our universe with everything else revolving around it.

We need to try and create a larger vision and purpose for ourselves in life in order to cope better with the pain. For many people, having a spiritual practice is a tremendous support.

---

* Radix Aconiti is a restricted substance in the UK.

Feeling that you are loved and on the right personal path in life is also very healing. None of us is perfect and it is not your fault that you are ill. Nevertheless it is your responsibility and no one else's to make the best of things. Even buying and reading this book demonstrates that you are trying to do this. I wholeheartedly encourage you to create some love and joy in your life so that pain is not the main focus.

CONCLUSION

The ideas and practices presented in this chapter are like cooking recipes. Just reading a cookbook without actually preparing the recipes can be entertaining, but it will not satisfy your hunger. The same is true for the suggestions offered here. I can tell you that these practices have been helpful for thousands of years but that will not satisfy your need, your hunger, unless you see for yourself. Therefore, the remedies on these pages need to be put into daily practice. They need to be cooked and baked in your experience. You don't need to do all of them. That is both impossible and unnecessary. Simply find one or two that intrigue you or make sense to try, and begin. Begin today. Nothing of worth has ever been accomplished without some effort.

FINDING A PRACTITIONER
OF CHINESE MEDICINE

Chinese medicine has grown enormously in the UK during the past 30 years. There are now at least 10 colleges that offer a professional training, some offering a university degree. Additionally, many excellent practitioners have come to the UK from the countries of East Asia.

Chinese medicine is a whole system of medicine with its own fundamental concepts and theories. It is not simply a technique. Previous knowledge or training in another system of medicine does not confer competence or knowledge in Chinese medicine. In order to get the most out of your therapy or treatment you should ensure that the practitioner is properly qualified and belongs to a professional body. Currently in the UK the onus is on the individual to check this situation. Members of these organisations are bound by a code of ethics and practice. They will have received an accredited level of training and will be covered by medical malpractice and public/products liability insurance.

When trying to find a good practitioner one of the best methods is word of mouth. Communication is also important if English is not their first language. It is fine to ask about their previous experience in treating your complaint. Many practitioners will be happy to talk on the phone or may offer a short introductory consultation so that you can assess whether you will feel comfortable working with them.

We have included Japanese traditions of herbal medicine (kanpo) and massage (shiatsu) in addition to Chinese. They originate from the same basic sources but have evolved differently in terms of style of practice.

The relevant professional bodies in the UK are:

Acupuncture
The British Acupuncture Council
63 Jeddo Road
London W12 9HQ
Tel: 020 8735 0400
Fax: 020 8735 0404
e-mail: info@acupuncture.org.uk
website: www.acupuncture.org.uk
Members have the initials MBAcC.

Chinese herbal medicine
The Register of Chinese Herbal Medicine
PO Box 400
Wembley, Middlesex
HA9 9NZ
Tel/Fax: 07000 790332
website: www.rchm.co.uk
Members have the initials MRCHM.

Japanese herbal medicine – Kanpo
The Kanpo Association
9a Ingatestone Rd
Brentwood, Essex
CM15 8AP
Tel: 01277 260080
Members have the initials KANPO.

Most members of the Kanpo Association are also members of
the RCHM. They are not bound by a code of ethics and practice
unless they are members of another professional body.

Shiatsu
The Shiatsu Society UK
Barber House
Storeys Bar Road
Fengate, Peterborough
PE1 5YS
Tel: 01733 758341
e-mail: shiatsu@graphic-scan.co.uk
Members have the initials MRSS.

Relevant bodies in other English-speaking countries are:

Australian Acupuncture & Chinese Medical Association (AACMA) is apparently the best professional organisation within Australia for patient contact.

AACMA
PO Box 5142
West End, Brisbane
Queensland
Australia 4101
Tel: +07 3846 5866
Fax: +07 3846 5276
Free Call: 1800 025 334
e-mail: aaca@eis.net.all
website: http://www2.eis.net.au/~aaca

The International Institute of Chinese Medicine and Acupuncture
PO Box 2246
19 Av Disandt-Fresnaye
Cape Town 8000
South Africa
Tel: 27 21 434 1654

LEARNING MORE ABOUT CHINESE MEDICINE

For more information about Chinese medicine in general, see:
Chinese Medicine: Acupuncture, Herbal Remedies, Nutrition, Qi Gong and Meditation by Tom Williams, Element Health Essentials.
This is a good basic introduction to the whole field of Chinese medicine for the layperson.

Acupuncture by Peter Mole, Element Books.
A simple and clear introduction to acupuncture for the layperson.

A Guide to Acupuncture by Peter Firebrace and Sandra Hill, Constable Books.
A comprehensive guide to acupuncture for the layperson with some illustrations and photographs.

Between Heaven and Earth: A Guide to Chinese Medicine by Harriet Beinfield and Efrem Korngold, Ballantine Books, New York.
This book is particularly good with regard to the more psychological and emotional aspects of Chinese medicine and has a good introduction to herbal medicine for the layperson.

Acupuncture in Practice edited by Hugh McPherson and Ted Kaptchuk, Churchill Livingston.
This is a book of case histories from the West. It illustrates the wide variety of styles and methods of practice of acupuncture by many well-known practitioners.

Chinese Herbal Medicine, a practical guide to the healing powers of herbs by Dr Guang Xu, Vermillion.
A good introduction to Chinese herbal medicine.

Japanese Acupuncture, a Clinical Guide, by Stephen Birch and Junko Ida, Paradigm Publications.
This book gives very good, clear details on moxibustion.

For more information on dietary therapy, see:
Healing with Wholefoods, Oriental Traditions and Modern Nutrition by Paul Pritchard, North Atlantic Books.
A comprehensive source book for both the layperson and the professional.

Helping Ourselves: A Guide to Traditional Chinese Food Energetics by Daverick Legget, Meridian Press.
This book is designed for ease of use with its clear layout and wall charts.

For more information on qi gong, see:
Stand Still Be Fit: The Way of Energy by Master Lam Kam Chuen, Gaia.
This is a very popular book and accompanying videotape which demonstrates qi gong exercises.

SUPPLIERS OF CHINESE HERBS

In the UK it is not possible to buy Chinese herbal medicines as a member of the public. You will need a prescription from a qualified Chinese herbalist. Some acupuncturists are able to prescribe traditional remedies or 'patents'. The suppliers we have listed here are members of CMAS – The Chinese Medicine Association of Suppliers. CMAS is a professional organisation which acts as a self-regulatory body to lobby in the interest of its members within the bounds of public safety. All members are subject to a code of practice.

Many of the members of CMAS have an excellent supply of books and other products relating to Chinese medicine/ acupuncture. Most if not all suppliers have a mail order service.

This list is by no means exhaustive: there are many other suppliers of acupuncture products and many shops which sell Chinese herbs. The acupuncture product suppliers are a good source should you wish to buy the seven star hammer mentioned in the chapter on home remedies. The herbal medicine shops may not be regulated.

Acumedic (MF Mei, Director)
101-105 Camden High Street
London NW1 7JN
Tel: 020 7388 5783 Fax: 020 7387 5766

Beijing Tong Ren Tang (Laurence Lo, Director)
124 Shaftesbury Avenue
London W1V 7DJ
Tel: 020 7287 0098 Fax: 020 7287 0068

China Medica (U Wiesman)
25 Lonsdale Close
London SE9 4HF
Tel: 020 8857 9777 Fax: 020 8480 2020

Chinese Medical Centre (Peter Ren, Director)
179 South Street, Romford
Essex RM1 1PS
Tel: 01708 756363 Fax: 01708 703015

East West Herbs (Robert Miller, Chief Executive)
Langston Priory Mews, Kingham
Oxfordshire OX7 6UP
Tel: 01608 658862 Fax: 01608 658816
e-mail: robert@eastwestherbs.co.uk

Great Wall (Barbara Zhang)
Unit 27, Riverside Works, Hertford Road
Barking IG11 8BN
Tel: 020 8591 6896 Fax: 020 8591 6891

Harmony Medical Distribution (Phil Choy)
629 High Road, Leytonstone
London E11 4PA
Tel: 020 8518 7337 Fax: 020 8556 5038
e-mail: Harmony@tcm.org.uk

Healthpack Ltd (Paul Skipworth)
Langston Priory Mews, Kingham
Oxfordshire OX7 6UP
Tel: 01608 658862 Fax: 01608 658816

Lotus
Priorsfield
Priory Forest Row
Sussex SH18 5HR
Tel: 01342 823053
Fax: 01342 826027

May Way UK
43 Waterside Trading Centre
Trumpers Way, Hanwell
Middlesex W7 2QD
Tel: 020 8893 6873
Fax: 020 8893 6874

Number One Herb Co
36 Bankhurst Road, Catford
London SE6 4XN
Tel/Fax: 020 8690 4840

Oxford Medical Supplies
Units 11 and 12 Horcott Industrial Estate
Fairford
Gloucestershire GL7 4LX
Tel: 0800 975 8000
Fax: 0800 975 8111

Shizhen TCM UK Ltd
50 Sandy Lane, Chorlton
Manchester M21 8TN
Tel: 0161 881 0088
Fax: 0161 881 0888

Tian Tiao Ltd
83 Sullivan Way
Elstree
Herts WD6 3DG
Tel: 020 8953 2320
Fax: 020 8953 3338

Naturally Chinese
PO Box 4584, Kiln Farm
Milton Keynes
Bucks MK13 9ZT
Tel: 0151 571 0407

CHINESE MEDICAL GLOSSARY

hinese medicine is a system unto itself. Its technical terms are uniquely its own and cannot be translated into the definitions of Western medicine without destroying their very fabric and logic. Ultimately, because Chinese medicine was created in the Chinese language, it is best understood in that language. Nevertheless, as Westerners trying to understand Chinese medicine, we must translate the technical terms of Chinese medicine into English words. If some of these technical translations sound peculiar at first and their meaning is not immediately transparent, this is because no equivalent concepts exist in everyday English.

In the past, some Western authors have erroneously translated technical Chinese medical terms using Western medical or at least quasi-scientific words in an attempt to make this system more easily understood by Western audiences. For instance, the words tonify and sedate are commonly seen in the Western Chinese medical literature even though, in the case of sedate, its meaning is the opposite to the Chinese understanding of the word *xie*. *Xie* means to drain off something which has pooled and accumulated. That accumulation is seen as something excess which should not be lingering where it is. Because it is accumulating somewhere where it shouldn't, it is impeding and obstructing whatever should be moving to and through that area. The word sedate comes from the Latin word *sedere*, to sit. Therefore, the word sedate means to make something sit still. In English, we get the word sediment from this same root. However, the Chinese *xie* means draining off that which is sitting somewhere erroneously. This mistranslation could be potentially misleading in terms of its clinical applications.

Therefore, in order to preserve the integrity of this system while still making it intelligible to English language readers, I have appended the following glossary of Chinese medical technical terms. The terms themselves are based on Nigel Wiseman's *English-Chinese Chinese-English Dictionary of Chinese Medicine* published by the Hunan Science and Technology Press in Changsha, Hunan, People's Republic of China in 1995. Dr Wiseman is, in my opinion, the greatest Western scholar in terms of the translation of Chinese medicine into English. As a Chinese reader myself, although I often find Wiseman's terms awkward-sounding at first, I also think they convey most accurately the Chinese understanding and logic of these terms.

Acquired essence: Essence manufactured out of the surplus of qi and blood in turn created out of the refined essence of food and drink

Acupoints: Those places on the channels and network vessels where qi and blood tend to collect in denser concentrations, and thus those places where the qi and blood in the channels are especially available for manipulation

Acupuncture: The regulation of qi flow by the stimulation of certain points located on the channels and network vessels achieved mainly by insertion of fine needles into these points

Bedroom taxation: Fatigue or vacuity due to excessive sex

Blood: The red-coloured fluids that flow in the vessels and nourishes and constructs the tissues of the body

Blood stasis: Also called dead blood, malign blood and dry blood, blood stasis is blood which is no longer moving through the vessels as it should. Instead it is precipitated in the vessels like silt in a river. Like silt, it then obstructs the free flow of the blood in the vessels and also impedes the production of new or fresh blood

Blood vacuity: Insufficient blood manifesting in diminished nourishment, construction and moistening of body tissues

Bowels: The hollow yang organs of Chinese medicine

Central qi: Also called the middle qi, this is synonymous with the spleen-stomach qi

Channels: The main routes for the distribution of qi and blood, but mainly qi

Clear: The pure or clear part of food and drink ingested that is then turned into qi and blood

Constructive qi: The qi that flows through the channels and nourishes and constructs the internal organs and body tissues

Counterflow: An erroneous flow of qi, usually upwards but sometimes horizontally as well

Damp heat: A combination of accumulated dampness mixed with pathological heat often associated with sores, abnormal vaginal discharges and some types of menstrual and body pain

Dampness: A pathological accumulation of body fluids

Decoction: A method of administering Chinese medicinals by boiling these medicinals in water, removing the dregs, and drinking the resulting medicinal liquid

Defensive qi: The yang qi that protects the exterior of the body from invasion by the environmental excesses

Depression: Stagnation and lack of movement, as in liver depression qi stagnation

Depressive heat: Heat due to enduring or severe qi stagnation which then transforms into heat

Drain: To drain off or away some pathological qi or substance from where it is replete or excess

Environmental excesses: A superabundance of wind, cold, dampness, dryness, heat or summer heat in the external environment which can invade the body and cause disease

Essence: A stored, very potent form of substance and qi, usually yin when compared to yang qi, but can be transformed into yang qi

External causes of disease: The six environmental excesses

Five phase theory: An ancient Chinese system of correspondences dividing up all of reality into five phases which then mutually engender and check each other according to definite sequences

Heat toxins: A particularly virulent and concentrated type of pathological heat often associated with purulence (*i.e.*, pus formation), sores and sometimes, but not always, malignancies

Hydrotherapy: Using various baths and water applications to treat and prevent disease

Impediment: A hindrance to the free flow of the qi and blood typically manifesting as pain and restriction in the range of movement of a joint or extremity

Internal causes of disease: The seven effects or emotions, namely, anger, joy (or excitement), sorrow, thought, fear, melancholy and fright

Lassitude of the spirit: A listless or apathetic effect or emotional demeanour due to obvious fatigue of the mind and body

Life gate fire: Another name for kidney yang or kidney fire, seen as the ultimate source of yang qi in the body

Magnet therapy: Applying magnets to acupuncture points to treat and prevent disease

Moxibustion: Burning the herb Artemisia Argyium on, over or near acupuncture points in order to add yang qi, warm cold or promote the movement of the qi and blood

Network vessels: Small vessels which form a net-like web ensuring the flow of qi and blood to all body tissues

Phlegm: A pathological accumulation of phlegm or mucus congealed from dampness or body fluids

Portals: Also called orifices, the openings of the sensory organs and the opening of the heart through which the spirit makes contact with the world outside

Qi: Activity, function, that which moves, transforms, defends, restrains and warms

Qi mechanism: The process of transforming yin substance controlled and promoted by the qi, largely synonymous with the process of digestion

Qi vacuity: Insufficient qi manifesting in diminished movement, transformation and function

Repletion: Excess or fullness, almost always pathological

Seven star hammer: A small hammer with needles embedded in its head used to stimulate acupoints without actually inserting needles

Spirit: The accumulation of qi in the heart which manifests as consciousness, sensory awareness and mental-emotional function

Stagnation: Non-movement of the qi, lack of free flow, constraint

Supplement: To add to or augment, as in supplementing the qi, blood, yin or yang

Turbid: The yin, impure, turbid part of food and drink that is sent downwards to be excreted as waste

Vacuity: Emptiness or insufficiency, typically of qi, blood, yin or yang

Vacuity cold: Obvious signs and symptoms of cold due to a lack or insufficiency of yang qix

Vacuity heat: Heat due to hyperactive yang in turn due to insufficient controlling yin

Vessels: The main routes for the distribution of qi and blood, but mainly blood

Viscera: The solid yin organs of Chinese medicine

Yang: In the body, function, movement, activity, transformation

Yang vacuity: Insufficient warming and transforming function giving rise to symptoms of cold in the body

Yin: In the body, substance and nourishment

Yin vacuity: Insufficient yin substance necessary to nourish, control and counterbalance yang activity

BIBLIOGRAPHY

CHINESE LANGUAGE SOURCES

Cheng Dan An Zhen Jiu Xuan Ji (*Cheng Dan-an's Selected Acupuncture and Moxibustion Works*), ed. by Cheng Wei-fen *et al.*, Shanghai Science and Technology Press, Shanghai, 1986

Chu Zhen Zhi Liao Xue (*A Study of Acupuncture Treatment*), Li Zhong-yu, Sichuan Science and Technology Press, Chengdu, 1990

Dong Yuan Yi Ji (*Dong-yuan's Collected Medical Works*), ed. by Bao Zheng-fei *et al.*, People's Health and Hygiene Press, Beijing, 1993

Han Ying Chang Yong Yi Xue Ci Hui (*Chinese-English Glossary of Commonly Used Medical Terms*), Huang Xiao-kai, People's Health and Hygiene Press, Beijing, 1982

Shang Hai Lao Zhong Yi Jing Yan Xuan Bian (*A Selected Compilation of Shanghai Old Doctors' Experiences*), Shanghai Science and Technology Press, Shanghai, 1984

Shi Yong Zhen Jiu Tui Na Zhi Liao Xue (*A Study of Practical Acupuncture, Moxibustion and Tui Na Treatments*), Xia Zhi-ping, Shanghai College of Chinese Medicine Press, Shanghai, 1990

Tan Zheng Lun (*Treatise on Phlegm Conditions*), Hou Tian-yin and Wang Chun-hua, People's Army Press, Beijing, 1989

Yi Zong Jin Jian (*The Golden Mirror of Ancestral Medicine*), Wu Qian *et al.*, People's Health and Hygiene Press, Beijing, 1985

Yu Xue Zheng Zhi (*Static Blood Patterns and Treatments*), Zhang Xue-wen, Shanxi Science and Technology Press, Xian, 1986

Zhen Jiu Da Cheng (*A Great Compendium of Acupuncture and Moxibustion*), Yang Ji-zhou, People's Health and Hygiene Press, Beijing, 1983

Zhen Jiu Xue (*A Study of Acupuncture and Moxibustion*), Qiu Mao-liang *et al.*, Shanghai Science and Technology Press, Shanghai, 1985

Zhen Jiu Yi Xue (*An Easy Study of Acupuncture and Moxibustion*), Li Shou-xian, People's Health and Hygiene Press, Beijing, 1990

Zhong Guo Min Jian Cao Yao Fang (*Chinese Folk Herbal Medicinal Formulas*), Liu Guang-rui and Liu Shao-lin, Sichuan Science and Technology Press, Chengdu, 1992

Zhong Guo Zhen Jiu Chu Fang Xue (*A Study of Chinese Acupuncture and Moxibustion Prescriptions*), Xiao Shao-qing, Ningxia People's Press, Yinchuan, 1986

Zhong Guo Zhong Yi Mi Fang Da Quan (*A Great Compendium of Chinese National Chinese Medical Secret Formulas*), ed. by Hu Zhao-ming, Literary Propagation Publishing Company, Shanghai, 1992

Zhong Yi Hu Li Xue (*A Study of Chinese Medical Nursing*), Lu Su- ying, People's Health and Hygiene Press, Beijing, 1983

Zhong Yi Lin Chuang Ge Ke (*Various Clinical Specialties in Chinese Medicine*), Zhang En-qin *et al.*, Shanghai College of Traditional Chinese Medicine Press, Shanghai, 1990

Zhong Yi Ling Yan Fang (Efficacious Chinese Medical Formulas), Lin Bin-zhi, Science and Technology Propagation Press, Beijing, 1991

ENGLISH LANGUAGE SOURCES

A Barefoot Doctor's Manual, revised and enlarged edition, Cloudburst Press, Mayne Isle, 1977

A Clinical Guide to Chinese Herbs and Formulae, Cheng Song-yu and Li Fei, Churchill Livingstone, Edinburgh, 1993

A Compendium of TCM Patterns and Treatments, Bob Flaws and Daniel Finney, Blue Poppy Press, Boulder, CO, 1996

A Comprehensive Guide to Chinese Herbal Medicine, Chen Ze-lin and Chen Mei-fang, Oriental Healing Arts Institute, Long Beach, CA, 1992

All About Arthritis, Derrick Brewerton, Harvard University Press, Cambridge, MA, 1992

The Dao of Healthy Eating According to Chinese Medicine, Bob Flaws, Blue Poppy Press, Boulder, CO, 1997

'Aspirin and Bleeding Peptic Ulcers in the Elderly', G. Faulkner *et al.*, *British Medical Journal*, Vol. 297, 1988, pp.1,311-13

A Handbook of Differential Diagnosis with Key Signs and Symptoms, Therapeutic Principles, and Guiding Prescriptions, Ou-yang Yi, trans. by C.S. Cheung, Harmonious Sunshine Cultural Center, San Francisco, 1987

Between Heaven and Earth: A Guide to Chinese Medicine, Harriet Beinfield and Efrem Korngold, Ballantine Books, New York, 1991

Bi-Syndromes or Rheumatic Disorders Treated by Traditional Chinese Medicine, L. Vangermeersch and Sun Pei-lin, SATAS, Belgium, 1994

Candida and Candidosis, F.C. Odds, University Park Press, Baltimore, 1979

Chinese-English Terminology of Traditional Chinese Medicine, Shuai Xue-zhong *et al.*, Hunan Science and Technology Press, Changsha, 1983

Chinese-English Manual of Common-used Prescriptions in Traditional Chinese Medicine, ed. by Ou Ming, Joint Publishing Co., Ltd., Hong Kong, 1989

Chinese Herbal Medicine: Formulas and Strategies, Dan Bensky and Randall Barolet, Eastland Press, Seattle, 1990

Chinese Herbal Medicine: Materia Medica, Dan Bensky and Andrew Gamble, second, revised edition, Eastland Press, Seattle, 1993

Chinese Herbal Teas: Simple, Proven Folk Formulas for Common Diseases and Promoting Health, Zong Xiao-fan and Gary Liscum, Blue Poppy Press, Boulder, CO, 1997

Chinese Medicinal Wines and Elixirs, Bob Flaws, Blue Poppy Press, Boulder, CO, 1995

Chinese Self-massage, The Easy Way to Health, Fan Ya-li, Blue Poppy Press, Boulder, CO, 1996

'Controlled Trial of Fasting and One-year Vegetarian Diet in Rheumatoid Arthritis', Kragh J. Kjeldsen *et al.*, *The Lancet*, Vol. 338, 1991, pp.899-902

'Detection of Chlamydia Trachomatis DNA in Joints of Reactive Arthritis Patients by Polymerase Chain Reaction', D. Gilroy Taylor-Robinson, *The Lancet*, Vol. 340, 1992, pp.81-2

'Diet for Rheumatoid Arthritis', L. G. Darlington and N. W. Ramsey, *The Lancet*, Vol. 338, 1991, p.1,209

'Drug-induced End Stage Renal Disease', P. Ronco and A. Flahault, *New England Journal of Medicine*, Vol. 331, No. 25, 1994, pp. 1711-12

English-Chinese Chinese-English Dictionary of Chinese Medicine, Nigel Wiseman, Hunan Science and Technology Press, Changsha, 1995

'Epidemiology of Adverse Reactions to Nonsteroidal Anti-inflammatory Drugs', J.C.P. Weber, *Advances in Inflammation*, Raven Press, NY, 1984

'Fasting and Vegan Diet in Rheumatoid Arthritis', L. Skoldstam, *Scandinavian Journal of Rheumatology*, Vol. 15, 1986, pp.219-23

'Food Allergy or Enterometabolic Disorder?', J.O. Hunter, *The Lancet*, Vol. 338, 1991, pp.495-6

Fundamentals of Chinese Acupuncture, Andrew Ellis, Nigel Wiseman and Ken Boss, Paradigm Publications, Brookline, MA, 1988

Fundamentals of Chinese Medicine, Nigel Wiseman and Andrew Ellis, Paradigm Publications, Brookline, MA, 1985

Glossary of Chinese Medical Terms and Acupuncture Points, Nigel Wiseman and Ken Boss, Paradigm Publications, Brookline, MA, 1990

Handbook of Chinese Herbs and Formulas, Him-che Yeung, self-published, LA, 1985

'Hepatotoxicity on Nonsteroidal Anti-inflammatory Drugs', R. Mordechai *et al.*, *The American Journal of Gastroenterology*, Vol. 87, 1992, pp.1,696-1,704

'NSAIDs and Osteoarthritis', P.M. Brooks *et al.*, *Journal of Rheumatology*, Vol. 9, 1982, pp.3-5

Oriental Materia Medica, a Concise Guide, Hong-yen Hsu, Oriental Healing Arts Institute, Long Beach, CA, 1986

Practical Traditional Chinese Medicine and Pharmacology: Clinical Experiences, Shang Xian-min *et al.*, New World Press, Beijing, 1990

Practical Traditional Chinese Medicine and Pharmacology: Herbal Formulas, Geng Jun-ying, *et al.*, New World Press, Beijing, 1991

'Prednisone Use in RA', Carol Potera, *Arthritis Today*, March-April, 1995, p. 8

Rheumatology in Chinese Medicine, Gérard Guillaume and Mach Chieu, Eastland Press, Seattle, 1996

Statements of Fact in Traditional Chinese Medicine, Bob Flaws, Blue Poppy Press, Boulder, CO

The Book of Jook: Chinese Medicinal Porridges, Bob Flaws, Blue Poppy Press, Boulder, CO, 1995

The Complete Book of Chinese Health and Healing, Daniel Reid, Shambhala, Boston, 1994

The English-Chinese Encyclopedia of Practical Traditional Chinese Medicine, ed. by Xuan Jia-sheng, Higher Education Press, Beijing, 1990

The Essential Book of Traditional Chinese Medicine, Liu Yan-chi, trans. by Fang Ting-yu and Chen Lai-di, Columbia University Press, NY, 1988

The History of Crime Against the Food Law: The Amazing Story of the National Food and Drug Law Intended to Protect the Health of the People Perverted to Protect Adulteration of Foods and Drugs, Harvey W. Wiley, self-published, Washington DC, 1929

The Merck Manual, 15th edition, ed. by Robert Berkow, Merck Sharp and Dohme Research Laboratories, Rahway, NJ, 1987

The Path, Laurie Beth Jones, Hyperion, NY

The Treatise on the Spleen and Stomach, Li Dong-yuan, trans. by Yang Shou-zhong, Blue Poppy Press, Boulder, CO, 1993

The Yeast Connection, William G. Crook, Vintage Books, Random House, NY, 1986

The Yeast Syndrome, John Parks Towbridge and Morton Walker, Bantam Books, Toronto, 1988

Traditional Medicine in Contemporary China, Nathan Sivin, University of Michigan, Ann Arbor, 1987

Zang Fu: The Organ Systems of Traditional Chinese Medicine, second edition, Jeremy Ross, Churchill Livingstone, Edinburgh, 1985

INDEX